Paediatric Skin and Wound Care

edited by
Richard White and Jacqueline Denyer

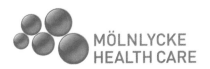
MÖLNLYCKE
HEALTH CARE

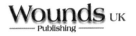
Wounds UK
—— Publishing ——

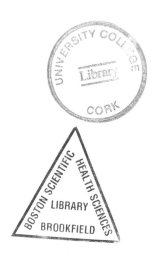

i 20206914

Wounds UK Publishing, Wounds UK Limited, Suite 3.1, 36 Upperkirkgate,
Aberdeen AB10 1BA

British Library Cataloguing-in-Publication Data
A catalogue record is available for this book

© Wounds UK Limited 2006
ISBN 0-9549193-6-X

Printed in the UK by Cromwell Press, Trowbridge, Wiltshire

CONTENTS

LIST OF CONTRIBUTORS

Elaine Bethell is Clinical Nurse Specialist, Tissue Viability, City Hospital, Birmingham.

Fiona Burton is Nurse Consultant in Tissue Viability, University Hospitals Coventry and Warwickshire NHS Trust.

Martyn Butcher is Clinical Nurse Specialist, Tissue Viability, Derriford Hospital, Plymouth.

Pat Coldicutt is Nurse Specialist, Stoma Care, Alder Hey Children's Hospital, Liverpool.

Jacqueline Denyer is Nurse Consultant for children with epidermolysis bullosa (EB), Great Ormond Street Hospital, London.

Krzysztof S Gebhardt is Clinical Nurse Specialist for Pressure Ulcer Prevention, St George's Healthcare NHS Trust, London.

Matthew Hardman is a Post-doctoral Research Associate, University of Manchester.

Valerie Irving is Unit Manager, Neonatal Unit, Liverpool Women's Hospital, Liverpool.

Kristina Soon is Chartered Clinical Psychologist for Dermatology, Great Ormond Street Hospital, London.

Rosemary Turnbull is Paediatric Dermatology Specialist Nurse, Chelsea and Westminster Hospital, London.

Richard White is a Clinical Research Consultant and Senior Research Fellow, Department of Tissue Viability, Aberdeen Royal Infirmary.

Jane Willock is Paediatric Nurse Practitioner, Children's Investigations Unit, University Hospital of Wales, Cardiff.

Trudie Young is Lecturer in Tissue Viability, School of Nursing and Midwifery, Glan Clwyd Hospital, Denbighshire.

FOREWORD

Few fields in nursing and medicine have advanced so rapidly in recent years as that of wound care. The very welcome specific growth in interest and knowledge of paediatric wound care has made this book both possible and necessary.

While a sound knowledge of wound care is necessary for so many branches of children's nursing, few paediatric nurses and doctors are able to regularly attend wound healing conferences to keep abreast of the many new insights and management advances in this complex field. These professionals will find that this book has collated, in a cohesive fashion, all that is best in paediatric skin and wound care. Beginning with an up-to-date summary of basic science as it pertains to the field, this book provides a structured and rigorous, yet accessible approach to the subject.

The scope of neonatal and paediatric medicine continues to expand, in particular the age of viability has dropped to 24 weeks. This success brings its own skin management challenges, and these issues are treated in a dedicated chapter

Management of rare disorders is well served, with one of the best resources available for nurses involved in the management of a child with epidermolysis bullosa (EB). This challenging condition often intimidates nurses unfamiliar with its particular demands, and herein is contained useful and vital advice for the first nurses to encounter a newborn with EB.

Those of us who work with children who have chronic wounds that require ongoing management, realise, that a happy, pain- and stress-free child will be more likely to comply with often demanding wound care regimens and will recover more quickly. It is welcome and appropriate to have chapters dealing with pain management and psychological aspects of wound care in this context.

This book has been written by practitioners acknowledged to be experts in their fields and, while accessible to non-specialist nurses, including community-based practitioners, it includes comprehensive reviews of the current evidence base and will be of great value to all nurses, regardless of their knowledge base and experience. The text can only help to raise awareness of the current depth of knowledge in this important field and, in so doing, improve outcomes for children and their families.

Alan Irvine MD, FRCPI, MRCP
Consultant Paediatric Dermatologist
Our Lady's Children's Hospital Crumlin
Dublin 12
Ireland

June 2006

CHAPTER 1

IN UTERO SKIN DEVELOPMENT

Matthew Hardman

The primary function of skin, the largest organ in the human body, is to provide a barrier between internal body structures and the environment. To better understand this role, the structure and development of human skin has been comprehensively documented (Holbrook, 1991). This has been followed by an explosion in the understanding of molecular characterisation of skin development, relying heavily on animal models. Indeed, correlation of molecular and ultrastructural data is leading to a comprehensive and detailed understanding of human skin development. This, in turn, is resulting in a rapidly expanding understanding of perturbed cutaneous development or maintenance, that is the molecular basis of a wide range of cutaneous disease states. The potential for gene therapy, a need to understand the immature skin of premature infants, the treatment of defects in wound healing, and a lucrative cosmetic industry are ensuring intense current interest in skin development. In particular, recent years have seen major advances in our understanding of epidermal stem cell biology (Barthel and Aberdam, 2005).

While this chapter is primarily focused on human *in utero* skin development, findings from animal models will be discussed where appropriate. Indeed, there is an ongoing need to relate an ever-expanding body of functional and molecular data from animal (predominantly mouse) models, with the more limited data available for human skin development.

The mature integument – structure and function

The integument, derived from the Latin *integumentum*, includes the skin, its appendages (hair, nails and glands), and a number of specialised epithelia. It is a highly evolved structure able to fulfil a diverse range of specialised functions. At the simplest level, the skin provides a physical barrier to desiccation and pathogens (Elias, 1983), protecting and cushioning underlying tissues. It also provides an environment for active immunological surveillance, and performs a wide range of sensory, thermoregulatory, respiratory, excretory, biosynthetic and socio-sexual functions (Kupper and Fuhlbrigge, 2004). The skin is a major biosynthetic organ producing large amounts of vitamin D and contains numerous melanocytes, which produce locally active pigmentation, protecting the body from potentially fatal ultraviolet radiation. The integument's role in body temperature regulation is particularly complex. In response to cold, dermal blood vessels contract; tiny muscles at the base of each follicle pull the hair erect trapping air to create a layer of insulation. Conversely, in response to heat, dermal blood vessels dilate and eccrine sweat glands excrete a mixture of water and salts which evaporate to cool the skin.

The skin is formed from the juxtaposition of two embryonic tissues, ectoderm (epidermis, hair, nails, skin glands) and mesoderm (connective tissue, vascular and lymphatics) during development. This gives rise to an outer epidermal layer in contact with an underlying basement membrane and an inner dermis (*Figure 1.1*). The epidermis and dermis are specialised for entirely different functions. The epidermis is a constantly renewing tissue that provides physical barrier function, via the specialised outermost layer, the stratum corneum. In contrast, the dermis provides support and nourishment.

Epidermal (keratinocyte) stem cells reside in the basal layer, a single proliferative layer in contact with the basement membrane (Watt, 2001; Fuchs *et al*, 2004). Stem cell division gives rise to new keratinocytes that are able to undergo limited proliferation before they migrate towards the skin surface and lose contact with the basement membrane. Once free, these cells move outwards and enter a non-reversible programme of terminal differentiation — a key feature of the keratinocyte life cycle. Keratinocytes are held together by specialised intercellular adhesion structures known as desmosomes and adherens junctions.

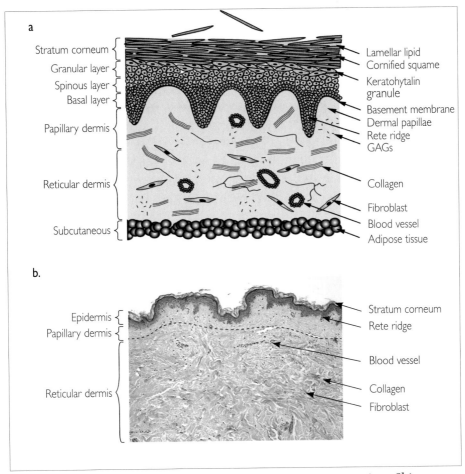

Figure 1.1: Adult skin structure. a) Diagrammatic representation. Skin comprises epidermis (yellow) and dermis (blue) separated by basement membrane. b) Histological section of adult human skin. Epidermal keratinocytes proliferate in the basal epidermal layer (mauve) and then move upwards undergoing a defined programme of differentiation. The dermis, which can be subdivided into papillary and reticular regions, is predominantly composed of fibroblasts and matrix. GAGs=dermal glycosaminoglycans

The proteins responsible for desmosome adhesion, cadherins, are differentially expressed through the epidermal layers. Recent evidence suggests a role for these different desmosomal cadherin isoforms in regulating epidermal differentiation (Hardman *et al*, 2005). Keratin filaments within the cell are anchored at desmosomes and provide the epidermis with a tough, fibrous network to help protect the skin from mechanical trauma (Fuchs, 1996). The progression of terminal differentiation as the keratinocyte migrates towards the skin surface is associated with changes in keratin isoform expression, followed by induction of cornified envelope precursor proteins and synthesis of non-polar lipids (Eckert *et al*, 1997). At the outermost periphery of the epidermis, keratinocytes undergo the final stages of terminal differentiation to form the stratum corneum (Candi *et al*, 2005). The epidermis is a continuously renewing tissue. Outermost cells are constantly shed (desquamation) and are replaced by keratinocytes from the lower epidermal layers. Epidermal turnover, or transit time, (from the basal layer keratinocyte to the outermost squame cell) varies between individual and body site, but is in the region of 28–35 days (Lindwall *et al*, 2006).

The basement membrane (dermal-epidermal interface) is anchored to the epidermis via integrin receptors, and to the dermis via anchoring fibrils. In humans, especially in the thickened palmoplantar skin of the hands and feet, the basement membrane is highly convoluted. Peg-like structures protrude from the dermis into the epidermis and vice versa, termed dermal papillae and rete ridges respectively (*Figure 1.1*). These structures are thought to provide a sheltered microenvironment for epidermal stem cells (keratinocytes) and transit amplifying cells (Cotsarelis *et al*, 1990). The hair follicle bulge has also been identified as an epidermal stem cell niche (Taylor *et al*, 2000). These undifferentiated cells are 'pluripotent'; that is, they have the potential to follow either an epidermal, or a follicular pathway. Hair follicle bulge-derived stem cells are able to undergo considerable horizontal migration into interfollicular epidermis. These stems cells are called upon during normal hair growth cycling, and provide a major source of new cells during cutaneous wound healing (Ito *et al*, 2005).

Below the basement membrane lies the dermis, a complex and dynamic connective tissue. The principal dermal cells, fibroblasts, sit in an intricate fibrillar extracellular matrix (ECM) composed of collagen, elastic fibres, fibronectin and numerous other matrix molecules (*Figure 1.1*). Collagen fibrils provide strength, while interconnecting networks of elastic fibres maintain structure. Dermal glycosaminoglycans (or GAGs), such as hyaluronic acid, impart massive water-holding capacity. This aqueous portion of the ECM allows rapid diffusion of nutrients, hormones and metabolites to the avascular epidermis, and provides turgor pressure, cushioning the skin and organs beneath against considerable compressive forces. GAG chains of varying size give rise to graded pores that differentially regulate the passage of signalling molecules and other molecular traffic (Keene *et al*, 1997). The activities of many enzymes and their inhibitors are regulated through interaction with ECM components, such as collagens. Collagens comprise a large family of matrix molecules, with over 25 subtypes. While adult skin collagen bundles are predominantly composed of type I collagen, other minor components, such as type V, play essential roles in fibrillogenesis and fibril stability (Kielty and Shuttleworth, 1997; Canty and Kadler, 2005), as evidenced by the large number of dermatological disorders resulting from collagen defects. In contrast to the epidermis, the dermis displays an outward to inward developmental gradient. Morphologically, the dermis can be divided into papillary and reticular regions. Deeper still, below the dermis, lies the hypodermis, a loose, connective tissue comprised of mostly adipose cells.

Epidermal development

The epidermis derives from a single layer of undifferentiated cuboidal embryonic ectodermal cells (*Figure 1.2*). During the late embryonic period, following periderm formation (Holbrook and Odland, 1975; see 'Periderm structure and function', *pp. 13–14*), the ectoderm stratifies giving rise to an intermediate cell layer (around 8 weeks) (Holbrook and Odland, 1980). Recent evidence suggests that this stratification is largely due to asymmetric cell division, perpendicularly orientated to the epithelial plane (Smart, 1970; Lechler and Fuchs, 2005). Functionally, intermediate layer cells are indistinguishable from those in the basal layer; both express keratins 8 and 18 (Moll *et al* 1982) and both proliferate (Bickenbach and Holbrook, 1987). This contrasts with the highly specialised mature epidermis, where suprabasal cell layers are highly differentiated. The embryonic/fetal transition (9–10 weeks) arguably marks the time of most important morphological change during *in utero* skin development. At the molecular level, this correlates with a developmental switch, signifying initiation of a terminal differentiation programme that will eventually give rise to adult epidermis (Dale *et al*, 1985). The switch is marked by the induction of keratins specifically associated with differentiating keratinocytes (keratin 1 and keratin 10) in intermediate layer cells (Dale *et al*, 1985; Fisher and Holbrook, 1987) (*Figure 1.3*). Basal layer keratinocytes now express the 'adult basal-marker' keratins (K5 and K14). Stratification and keratin induction are regional in both animal models and the human infant (Hoyes, 1968; Hardman *et al*, 1998; 1999). The basement membrane undergoes major changes in this period. Anchoring filaments and hemidesmosomes become more abundant (Smith *et al*, 1982). Hemidesmosomal integrin receptors switch from peri-cellular expression to basement membrane localisation (Hertle *et al*, 1991). Basal cells become polarised and the cell-cell keratinocyte adhesion junctions, desmosome and adherens junctions relocate to lateral and apical membranes (Hentula *et al*, 2001).

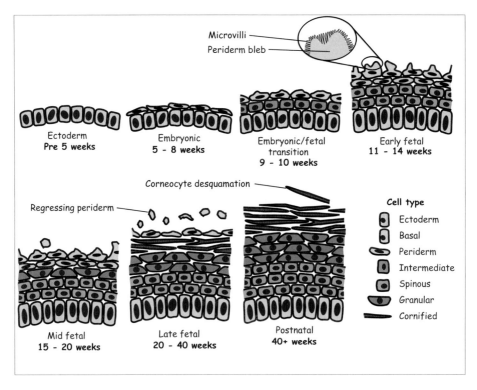

Figure 1.2: Schematic diagram of the key stages of ectodermal/epidermal development, from a single layer of undifferentiated ectoderm (5–8 weeks) to a multilayered stratified differentiated epithelia (40 weeks). Periderm differentiates and becomes functional (indicated by belbbing and formation of microvilli) in the early fetal period, then regresses during the late fetal period. Epidermal terminal differentiation culminates in formation of the stratum corneum and acquisition of barrier function during the late fetal period

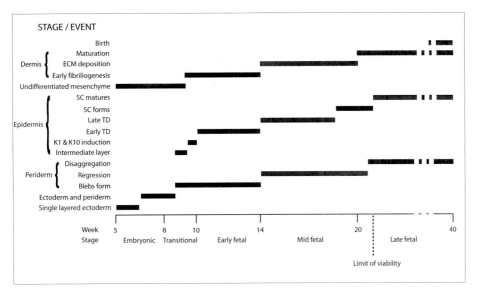

Figure 1.3: A detailed temporal representation of the key stages and events in the formation of dermis, epidermis and periderm. ECM = extracellular matrix, SC = stratum corneum, TD = terminal differentiation

The embryonic/fetal transition period can be reproduced in keratinocyte culture models, where induction of terminal differentiation is dependent on complex signalling events (Dotto, 1999; Watt, 2001). The epidermis contains a calcium gradient, and changes in calcium levels as cells transit through the tissue are believed to be instrumental in regulating appropriate gene expression. Of note, the S100 family of differentially expressed EF-hand motif proteins are emerging as important mediators of calcium-associated signal transduction (Eckert *et al*, 2004). The S100 family of proteins bind calcium; they play a role in cell-cell interactions and in epidermal disease as they are over-expressed in wound healing, inflammation, psoriasis and skin cancer (McNutt, 1998; Eckert *et al*, 2004).

Specialised non-keratinocyte epidermal cells appear during the late embryonic period (Holbrook and Odland, 1975; Smith *et al*, 1982). These are neural-crest derived melanocytes (*Chapter 2*); they begin to populate the epidermis during week seven. However, pigment production initiates much later, at around 14 weeks, and pigment is only transferred to keratinocytes during the mid- to late-fetal period. Similarly, while Langerhans (mesenchymally-derived dendritic) cells are found in the epidermis as early as week six, they only acquire antigen presenting function at, or after birth. Specialist mechanoreceptor Merkel cells are the last major epidermal cell type to appear at eight weeks in palmar/plantar epidermis. Merkel cells later localise to epidermal ridges and are subsequently detected in the dermis (Moll et al, 1986).

From the early- to mid-fetal period (11–20 weeks), the epidermis undergoes more subtle changes. Additional epidermal layers are added and a distinctive spinous layer forms (Figure 1.2). It is during this period that appendages appear and mature (see 'Appendage formation', pp. 12–13). The last major change in epidermal morphology, the formation of the stratum corneum or keratinisation, coincides with the beginning of the late fetal period (20–24 weeks) (Hardman et al, 1999) over most of the body. Stratum corneum formation is highly regional; it is first detected at 18 weeks when it is associated with more mature hair follicles in the head region (Holbrook and Odland, 1978), and over the nail bed (Holbrook and Odland, 1980). In humans, stratum corneum formation is complex, influenced by both follicles and specialised skin initiation regions, and moving fronts of epidermal terminal differentiation identified in animal models (Hardman et al, 1998; 1999) (Figure 1.4). The stratum corneum has a highly specialised structure of corneocytes, or squames (end-stage keratinocytes), with an impermeable ceramide (lipid) encased cornified envelope (Nemes and Steinert, 1999) embedded in a highly ordered non-polar lipid matrix (Wertz, 2000). This structure, which is virtually impenetrable to water and other hydrophobic molecules, provides a formidable cutaneous barrier function. Hence, infants who are born on or around the limit of viability (presently 22 weeks gestation), are susceptible to dehydration and/or infection as they have little or no mature stratum corneum water permeability barrier function (Hammarlund and Sedin 1979; Wilson and Maibach, 1980; Hardman et al, 1999; see also Chapter 2).

The stratum corneum is formed from numerous protein components synthesised during late terminal differentiation. The formation of the cornified cell envelope is initiated by enzymic crosslinking of the early scaffold proteins envoplakin, periplakin and involucrin at the plasma membrane (DiColandrea et al, 2000). Next, aggregates of cross-bridging proteins and the major envelope precursor loricrin form; this is mediated by the cytoplasmic transglutaminase-3 enzyme. These aggregates are then directly incorporated into the cornified envelope (Kalinin et al, 2001). More specialised cornified envelope proteins include the keratin filament-binding protein filaggrin (Simon et al, 1996), and the late cornified envelope (LCE) proteins, which are expressed in the epidermis just prior to the barrier formation (Zhao and Elder, 1997; Marshall *et al*, 2001; Jackson *et al*, 2005). These late incorporated proteins may confer subtle tissue and body-site specific changes in envelope properties and barrier quality. The extracellular lipid envelope and lipid matrix are derived from abundant stratum granulosum (granular layer) synthesised lamellar bodies. The contents of these sub-cellular organelles are non-polar lipids and lipid-processing enzymes; they are extruded into the intercorneocyte space and re-arranged into the lamellar sheets characteristic of mature stratum corneum (Chapman and Walsh, 1989; Elias *et al*, 1998; Nemes *et al*, 1999; Behne *et al*, 2000).

In adult skin, the majority of epidermal barrier function has been suggested to reside in the region of the stratum corneum, known as the stratum compactum (Bowser and White 1985; *Chapter 2*). However, recent animal models indicate additional levels of complexity and redundancy. For example, mice lacking claudin-1 (a major tight junction component present in the living epidermal layers) die at birth from barrier defects (Furuse *et al*, 2002), while mice lacking loricrin (the most abundant cornified envelope precursor) are viable with little barrier abnormality (Koch *et al*, 2000). Permeability assays, which measure an extremely early stage in barrier formation, show that barrier forms regionally in the human infant between 20 and 24 weeks gestation (Hardman *et al*, 1999) (*Figure 1.4*). The barrier appears at hair follicles and at non-follicular initiation sites, then propagates outwards across the body. In the human infant, the barrier initiates on the head, face and neck at 18–20 weeks, then over several weeks propagates across the epidermis to cover the abdomen and the back (Hardman *et al*, 1999). The barrier forms slightly after initial stratum corneum formation, reflecting several maturational events in the newly-formed cornified layer. Specifically, barrier formation exactly correlates with adoption of a flattened electron-dense morphology in the single layer of corneocytes. Deposition of additional stratum corneum layers leads to further barrier acquisition (also termed barrier maturation), as measured by an evaporimeter (Nilsson, 1977) up to 32 weeks (Hammarlund and Sedin, 1979; Wilson and Maibach, 1980; Harpin and Rutter, 1983).

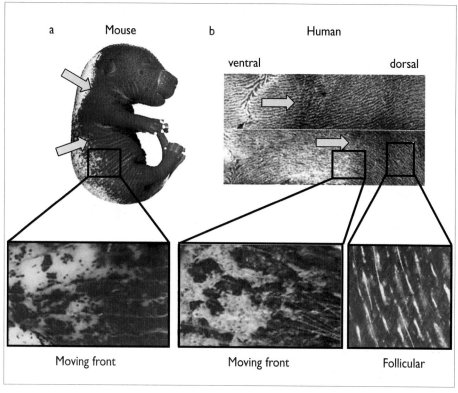

Figure 1.4: The epidermal permeability barrier is induced regionally in the human infant between 20 and 24 weeks. a) Our functional barrier assays, developed in rodents, identify novel regions of barrier initiation (termed initiation sites, white areas), barrier then propagates across the epidermis as moving fronts (arrows; high power boxout). A blue result from a dye exclusion assay indicates lack of barrier. b) At 22 weeks a strip of skin from the torso of a pre-term infant has distinct barrier positive regions (white areas) that are propagated around the body as a ventral to dorsal wave (arrows). Note the similarity between the mouse and human moving fronts of barrier acquisition at high magnification. In humans, prior to the barrier front, follicles act as initiation sites (far right boxout)

Dermal development

Prior to eight weeks (the early embryonic period), the dermis is an indistinct primordial dermal mesenchyme. The sub-epidermal surface is cellular and devoid of detectable fibrous material (Smith and Holbrook, 1986). During these early cellular stages of dermal development, the dermis and epidermis are separated by a simple basal lamina. As early as week five, collagen IV and laminin deposition indicate early steps towards basement membrane formation (Fine _et al_, 1984; Smith _et al_, 1986). At the beginning of the embryonic/fetal transition period, dermal cells begin to differentiate, following several different lineages, and the dermal-subdermal boundary becomes defined by vascular development (appearance of endothelial cells) (Smith and Holbrook, 1986). The predominant dermal cell, the fibroblast, appears at around week nine. The main role of fibroblasts is secretory, and their arrival correlates with major acceleration in the rate of deposition of fibrous material and matrix in the dermis (Smith and Holbrook, 1986; Smith _et al_, 1986) (_Figure 1.3_). Hence, the early fetal period is characterised by increasing dermal matrix deposition. Deposited matrix proteins are first arranged into small fibrils of around 20 nm in diameter. Fibril size steadily increases to form long dense fibres of 60 nm diameter or greater. This period is marked by massive dermal expansion (a greater than ten-fold increase in thickness during development), and dermal stratification. Expansion leads to a decrease in fibroblast density, and the resulting gaps are filled by new fibrils and other newly-synthesised matrix components.

By the beginning of the mid-fetal period, adiopocytes (connective tissue cells specialised for the synthesis and storage of fat) are present, likely acting as a source of growth factors (Williams _et al_, 1988). By the late-fetal period, the dermis contains more specialised cell types such as macrophages, pericytes and mast cells. Although morphologically the developing dermis now closely resembles adult dermis, there are major differences at the molecular level. For example, developing dermis is rich in type III collagen fibres, whereas adult dermis is predominately composed of type I collagen (Kielty and Shuttleworth, 1997). It is interesting to note that pathways regulating development are most likely re-used in the cutaneous healing process, where wound granulation tissue contains high levels of collagen III. Dermal development, in common with epidermal differentiation, is highly regional with large body-site specific variation in dermal thickness, composition and developmental stage (Aktan _et al_, 1999).

Appendage formation

Skin appendages are highly specialised, morphologically complex structures that fulfil diverse roles both during development and in adulthood (Chuong and Noveen, 1999). Skin development involves early juxtaposition of mesodermal and ectodermal tissues. A vast body of experimental work, predominantly from the chick, shows that cross-talk between the two tissues is absolutely necessary for formation of skin appendages such as hair, nails and glands (reviewed in Sengel, 1990). The initial signal to 'make an appendage' comes from the dermis, and the type of appendage that forms is governed by the dermis. However, morphologically, the earliest events in follicle formation involve the ectoderm. The first sign of an appendage is the appearance of an embryonic ectoderm placode, a cluster of elongated cells that will form the appendage. The placode then signals back to the mesenchyme, causing mesenchymal cells to cluster beneath the placode. A series of controlled morphogenic changes lead to formation of an ectodermal germ and dermal papilla. At this primordial stage, hairs and other appendages, such as glands, appear identical. Subsequent development will generate each unique appendage structure. Epithelial-mesenchymal signalling is complex. Formation of appendages involves complex signalling events, involving cross-talk and interaction between large groups of signalling molecules, including members of the notch, sonic hedgehog (a family of growth factors involved in cell-cell communication during development), and Wnt pathways (secreted proteins that are essential for many developmental and physiological processes, including cell to cell interactions during embryogenesis) (Cadigan and Liu, 2006) that specify follicle spacing, follicle type, morphogenesis and differentiation and, in later life, regulate cycling and function. Early morphogenesis correlates with marked changes in cell adhesion proteins, such as E- and P-cadherin (Byrne *et al*, 2003).

The most conspicuous feature of the early-fetal period in humans is the appearance of hair germs at 12 weeks. The earliest hair follicles form on the scalp, and subsequent follicles are reported to appear in a cephalocaudal direction, moving around the body as a wave (Holbrook and Odland, 1978). By the late-fetal period, the fetus is thinly covered by lanugo, which will later be replaced by fine vellus hair. Sebaceous glands are the first type to appear, at around 16 weeks, in conjunction with hair development (Sato *et al*, 1977). Eccrine glands are next to form at the beginning of the late-fetal period, followed by apocrine glands which only become active at around 34 weeks.

Periderm structure and function

The periderm, a transient embryonic ectoderm-derived layer, forms during the embryonic period prior to epidermal stratification (*Figure 1.2*). In contrast to other cutaneous tissues, the role of periderm during development is somewhat uncertain. Its primary function is thought to be the provision of an interface between embryo and amniotic fluid for much of *in utero* development. However, the exact function probably varies with the developmental stage. Initially, periderm appears to have an interactive role with amniotic fluid. After a short proliferative period, periderm cells flatten considerably and undergo morphological changes, including formation of outer cell surface blebs with numerous microvilli and intercellular transport vesicles (*Figure 1.3*). The enormous resultant increase in surface area has led to speculation that periderm has an absorptive or an excretory role (Holbrook and Odland, 1975; Hoyes, 1968). Indeed, the amniotic fluid may be a key source of epidermal nutrients prior to formation of the mature dermal capillary networks.

Periderm develops and differentiates in tandem with the epidermis, finally dissociating late in gestation as the stratum corneum forms (Saathoff *et al*, 2004) (*Figure 1.2*). Dissociated periderm is a major component of vernix caseosa, the slippery white epidermal covering that acts as a lubricant and moisturiser during birth, and as a barrier and site of innate defence immediately after birth (Visscher *et al*, 2005). During late gestation, regressing periderm is thought to form a barrier between the delicate underlying epidermis and the amniotic fluid. This is supported by the presence of tight junctions between periderm cells (Morita *et al*, 1998; Pummi *et al*, 2001). Periderm dissociation is the last major step in *in utero* skin development. Epidermal and peridermal differentiation are surprisingly similar; both tissues form cornified envelopes (Akiyama *et al*, 1999; Lee *et al*, 1999), again indicating a protective role. It is interesting that periderm dissociates in tandem with epidermal stratum corneum formation, or acquisition of epidermal barrier at approximately 22–25 weeks, the time when an absorptive function would become redundant. In humans, the periderm can persist until birth, leading to the rare condition, collodion baby (Sandler and Hashimoto, 1998). Invariably in these neonates, the underlying epidermis is also abnormal, leading to a life-threatening lack of cutaneous barrier.

Summary

Birth marks the most extreme change in environment we are ever likely to experience. As neonates, we are instantaneously moved from the warm, aseptic liquid *in utero* setting that has been home for many months, into a harsh, dry, terrestrial environment. As outlined in this chapter, the developing skin undergoes major morphological change that includes acquisition of epidermal barrier structures, appendages and dermal matrix that comprise this highly specialised, dynamic adult organ. That these preparatory events necessary for survival in a desiccating atmosphere occur in an entirely aqueous environment is particularly impressive. The importance of functional skin is outlined by the extensive water balance and infection problems experienced by infants born on, or around, the limit of viability. Major advances in our understanding of the molecular regulation of cutaneous biology are bringing us ever closer to comprehensive therapies for the treatment of prematurity and a wide range of dermatological conditions, and are opening up the possibilities of scar-free healing and complete tissue regeneration.

References

Aktan M, Buyukmumcu M, Seker M *et al* (1999) Morphometric analyses of the development of dermis in human fetuses. *Kaibogaku Zasshi* 74: 639–42

Akiyama M, Smith LT, Yoneda K *et al* (1999) Periderm cells form cornified cell envelope in their regression process during human epidermal development. *J Invest Dermatol* 112: 903–9

Barthel R, Aberdam D (2005) Epidermal stem cells. *J Eur Acad Dermatol Venereol* 19(4): 405–13

Behne M, Uchida Y, Seki T *et al* (2000) Omega-hydroxylceramides are required for corneocyte lipid envelope (CLE) formation and normal epidermal permeability barrier function. *J Invest Dermatol* **114**: 185–92

Bickenbach JR, Holbrook KA (1987) Label-retaining cells in human embryonic and fetal epidermis. *J Invest Dermatol* **88**: 42–6

Bowser PA, White RJ (1985) Isolation, barrier properties and lipid analysis of stratum compactum, a discrete region of stratum corneum. *Br J Dermatol* **12**: 1–14

Byrne C, Hardman M, Nield K (2003) Covering the limb — formation of the integument. *J Anat* **202**(1): 113–23

Butcher M, White R (2005) The structure and functions of the skin. In: White R, ed. *Skin Care in Wound Management: Assessment, prevention and treatment*. Wounds UK, Aberdeen

Cadigan KM, Liu Y (2006) Wnt signalling; complexity at the surface. *J Cell Sci* **119**(3): 395–402

Candi E, Schmidt R, Melino G (2005) The cornified envelope: a model of cell death in the skin. *Nat Rev Mol Cell Biol* **6**: 328–40

Canty EG, Kadler KE (2005) Procollagen trafficking, processing and fibrillogenesis. *J Cell Sci* **118**(7): 1341–53

Chapman SJ, Walsh A (1989) Membrane-coating granules are acidic organelles which possess proton pumps. *J Invest Dermatol* **93**(4): 466–70

Chuong CM, Noveen A (1999) Phenotypic determination of epithelial appendages: genes, developmental pathways, and evolution. *J Invest Dermatol Symp Proc* **4**: 307–11

Cotsarelis G, Sun TT, Lavker RM (1990) Label-retaining cells reside in the bulge area of pilosebaceous unit: implications for follicular stem cells, hair cycle, and skin carcinogenesis. *Cell* **61**: 1329–37

Dale BA, Holbrook KA, Kimball JR, Hoff M, Sun TT (1985) Expression of epidermal keratins and filaggrin during human fetal skin development. *J Cell Biol* **101**: 1257–69

DiColandrea T, Karashima T, Maatta A, Watt FM (2000) Subcellular distribution of envoplakin and periplakin: insights into their role as precursors of the epidermal cornified envelope. *J Cell Biol* **151**: 573–86

Dotto GP (1999) Signal transduction pathways controlling the switch between keratinocyte growth and differentiation. *Crit Rev Oral Biol Med* **10**: 442–57

Eckert RL, Crish JF, Robinson NA (1997) The epidermal keratinocyte as a model for the study of gene regulation and cell differentiation. *Physiol Rev* **77**(2): 397–424

Eckert RL, Broome AM, Ruse M *et al* (2004) S100 proteins in the epidermis. *J Invest Dermatol* **123**: 23–33

Elias PM (1983) Epidermal lipids, barrier function and desquamation. *J Invest Dermatol* **80**: 44–9

Elias PM, Cullander C, Mauro T *et al* (1998) The secretory granular cell: the outermost granular cell as a specialized secretory cell. *J Invest Dermatol Symp Proc* **3**: 87–100

Fine JD, Smith LT, Holbrook KA, Katz SI (1984) The appearance of four basement membrane zone antigens in developing human fetal skin. *J Invest Dermatol* **83**: 66–9

Fisher C, Holbrook KA (1987) Cell surface and cytoskeletal changes associated with epidermal stratification and differentiation in organ cultures of embryonic human skin. *Dev Biol* **119**: 231–41

Fuchs E (1993) Epidermal differentiation and keratin gene expression. *J Cell Sci* (Suppl) **17**: 197–208

Fuchs E (1996) The cytoskeleton and disease: genetic disorders of intermediate filaments. *Ann Rev Genet* **30**: 197–231

Fuchs E, Tumbar T, Guasch G (2004) Socializing with the neighbors: stem cells and their niche. *Cell* **116**: 769–78

Furuse M, Hata M, Furuse K, Yoshida Y, Haratake A, Sugitani Y *et al* (2002) Claudin-based tight junctions are crucial for the mammalian epidermal barrier: a lesson from claudin-1-deficient mice. *J Cell Biol* **156**: 1099–11

Hammarlund K, Sedin G (1979) Transepidermal water loss in newborn infants: III. Relation to gestational age. *Acta Paediatr Scand* **68**: 795–801

Hardman MJ, Moore L, Ferguson MWJ, Byrne C (1999) Barrier formation in the human fetus is patterned. *J Invest Dermatol* **113**: 1106–14

Hardman MJ, Sisi P, Banbury DN, Byrne C (1998) Patterned acquisition of barrier function during development. *Development* **128**: 1541–52

Hardman MJ, Liu K, Avilion AA, Merritt A *et al* (2005) Desmosomal cadherin misexpression alters beta-catenin stability and epidermal differentiation. *Mol Cell Biol* **25**: 969–78

Harpin VA, Rutter N (1983) Barrier properties of the newborn infant's skin. *J Pediatr* **102**: 419–25

Hentula M, Peltonen J, Peltonen S (2001) Expression profiles of cell-cell and cell-matrix junction proteins in developing human epidermis. *Arch Dermatol Res* **293**: 259–67

Hertle MD, Adams JC, Watt FM (1991) Integrin expression during human epidermal development in vivo and in vitro. *Development* **112**: 193–206

Holbrook KA (1991) Structure and function of the developing human skin. In: Goldsmith LA, ed. *Physiology, Biochemistry and Molecular Biology of the Skin*. 2nd edn. Oxford University Press, New York: 63–110

Holbrook KA, Odland GF (1975) The fine structure of developing human epidermis: light, scanning, and transmission electron microscopy of the periderm. *J Invest Dermatol* 65: 16–38

Holbrook KA, Odland GF (1978) Structure of the human fetal hair canal and initial hair eruption. *J Invest Dermatol* 71: 385–90

Holbrook KA, Odland GF (1980) Regional development of the human epidermis in the first trimester embryo and the second trimester fetus (ages related to the time of amniocentesis and fetal biopsy). *J Invest Dermatol* 74: 161–8

Hoyes AD (1968) Electron microscopy of the surface layer (periderm) of human fetal skin. *J Anat* 103: 321–36

Ito M, Liu Y, Yang Z, Nguyen J *et al* (2005) Stem cells in the hair follicle bulge contribute to wound repair but not to homeostasis of the epidermis. *Nat Med* 11: 1351–4

Jackson B, Tilli CL, Hardman M *et al* (2005) Late cornified envelope family in differentiating epithelia — response to calcium and ultraviolet irradiation. *J Invest Dermatol* 124: 1062–70

Kalinin A, Marekov LN, Steinert PM (2001) Assembly of the epidermal cornified cell envelope. *J Cell Sci* 114: 3069–70

Keene DR, Marinkovich MP, Sakai LY (1997) Immunodissection of the connective tissue matrix in human skin. *Microsc Res Tech* 38: 394–406

Kielty CM, Shuttleworth CA (1997) Microfibrillar elements of the dermal matrix. *Microsc Res Tech* 38: 413–27

Koch PJ, de Viragh PA, Scharer E, Bundman D, Longley MA, Bickenbach J *et al* (2000) Lessons from loricrin-deficient mice: compensatory mechanisms maintaining skin barrier function in the absence of a major cornified envelope protein. *J Cell Biol* 151: 389–400

Kupper TS, Fuhlbrigge RC (2004) Immune surveillance in the skin: mechanisms and clinical consequences. *Nat Rev Immunol* 4: 211–22

Lechler T, Fuchs E (2005) Asymmetric cell divisions promote stratification and differentiation of mammalian skin. *Nature* 437: 275–80

Lee SC, Lee JB, Kook JP *et al* (1999) Expression of differentiation markers during fetal skin development in humans: immunohistochemical studies on the precursor proteins forming the cornified cell envelope. *J Invest Dermatol* 112: 882–6

Lindwall G, Hsieh E, Misell LM *et al* (2006) Heavy water labelling of keratin as a non-invasive biomarker of skin turnover in vivo. *J Invest Dermatol* Feb: E-publication ahead of print

McNutt NS (1998) The S100 family of multipurpose calcium-binding proteins. *J Cutan Pathol* 25(10): 521–9

Marshall D, Hardman MJ, Nield KM, Byrne C (2001) Differentially expressed late constituents of the epidermal cornified envelope. *Proc Natl Acad Sci USA* **98**(23): 13031–6

Moll I, Moll R, Franke WW (1986) Formation of epidermal and dermal Merkel cells during human fetal skin development. *J Invest Dermatol* **87**: 779–87

Moll R, Moll I, Wiest W (1982) Changes in the pattern of cytokeratin polypeptides in epidermis and hair follicles during skin development in human fetuses. *Differentiation* **23**: 170–8

Morita K, Itoh M, Saitou M *et al* (1998) Subcellular distribution of tight junction-associated proteins (occludin, ZO-1, ZO-2) in rodent skin. *J Invest Dermatol* **110**: 862–6

Nemes Z, Steinert PM (1999) Bricks and mortar of the epidermal barrier. *Exp Mol Med* **31**: 5–19

Nemes Z, Marekov LN, Fésüs L, Steinert PM (1999) A novel function for transglutaminase 1: attachment of long-chain omega-hydroxyceramides to involucrin by ester bond formation. *Proc Natl Acad Sci USA* **96**: 8402–7

Nilsson GE (1977) Measurement of water exchange through the skin. *Med Biol Eng Comput* **15**: 209–18

Pummi K, Malminen M, Aho H *et al* (2001) Epidermal tight junctions: ZO-1 and occludin are expressed in mature, developing, and affected skin and in vitro differentiating keratinocytes. *J Invest Dermatol* **117**: 1050–8

Saathoff M, Blum B, Quast T, Kirfel G, Herzog V (2004) Simultaneous cell death and desquamation of the embryonic diffusion barrier during epidermal development. *Exp Cell Res* **299**: 415–26

Sandler B, Hashimoto K (1998) Collodion baby and lamellar ichthyosis. *J Cutan Pathol* **25**(2): 116–21

Sato S, Hiraga K, Nishijima A, Hidano A (1977) Neonatal sebaceous glands: fine structure of sebaceous and dendritic cells. *Acta Derm Venereol* **57**: 279–87

Sengel P (1990) Pattern formation in skin development. *Int J Dev Biol* **34**: 33–50

Simon M, Haftek M, Sebbag M *et al* (1996) Evidence that filaggrin is a component of the cornified cell envelope in human planter epidermis. *J Biochem* **317**: 173–7

Smart IH (1970) Variation in plane of cell cleavage during the process of stratification in mouse epidermis. *Br J Dermatol* **82**: 276–82

Smith LT, Holbrook KA, Byers PH (1982) Structure of the dermal matrix during development and in the adult. *J Invest Dermatol* **79**: S93–S104

Smith LT, Holbrook KA (1986) Embryogenesis of the dermis in human skin. *Pediatr Dermatol* **3**: 271–80

Smith LT, Holbrook KA, Madri JA (1986) Collagen types I, III, and V in human embryonic and fetal skin. *Am J Anat* **175**: 507–21

Taylor G, Lehrer MS, Jensen PJ, Sun TT, Lavker RM (2000) Involvement of follicular stem cells in forming not only the follicle but also the epidermis. *Cell* **102**: 451–61

Visscher MO, Narendran V, Pickens WL *et al* (2005) Vernix caseosa in neonatal adaptation. *J Perinatol* **25**: 440–6

Watt FM (2001) Stem cell fate and patterning in mammalian epidermis. *Curr Opin Genet Dev* **11**: 410–17

Wertz PW (2000) Lipids and barrier function of the skin. *Acta Derm Venereol Suppl* (Stockh) **208**: 7–11

Williams ML, Hincenbergs M, Holbrook KA (1988) Skin lipid content during early fetal development. *J Invest Dermatol* **91**: 263–8

Wilson DR, Maibach HI (1980) Transepidermal water loss in vivo: premature and term infants. *Biol Neonate* **37**: 180–5

Zhao XP, Elder JT (1997) Positional cloning of novel skin-specific genes from the human epidermal differentiation complex. *Genomics* **45**: 250–8

CHAPTER 2

THE STRUCTURE AND FUNCTIONS OF THE SKIN: PAEDIATRIC VARIATIONS

Richard White and Martyn Butcher

The skin is the largest organ of the body providing, in the adult, about 10% of the body mass and covering an area of almost 2 square metres. Human skin has evolved to help us regulate heat and water loss while acting as a barrier to the invasion of microorganisms and harmful chemicals. This chapter considers the detailed anatomy of each of the skin's layers, together with an overview of the major physiological and metabolic functions. It provides an insight into structure and function of children's skin that will help the clinician understand the mechanisms of damage that might occur, and, the rationale for preventive and therapeutic interventions.

In gross terms, the skin comprises two major tissue layers, the cellular epidermis and the largely acellular dermis. Associated with these layers are a variety of appendages, such as hair follicles, sweat glands, nerve endings and blood vessels.

The epidermis

The epidermis is the superficial cellular layer of the skin (*Figure 2.1*). The development of the structures of the epidermis is proportional to the gestational age of the infant. In premature infants, the epidermis is 20–25 mm thick, compared to 40–50 mm in full-term neonates, and > 50 mm in infants and children. The palmar and plantar surfaces are recognised as being 'extra protective', designed for walking and handling; this thickened tissue is the end product of epidermal cell differentiation. While these areas are evident in the adult, even the palmo-plantar skin of the full-term infant is already thickened in preparation for future physical wear and tear. The epidermis has no direct blood supply, it receives all of its nutrients and oxygen by diffusion from the vascular network in the superficial (papillary) dermis. The epidermis comprises a number of cell layers (*Figure 2.2*), each being a stage in the differentiation process of the major epidermal cell — the keratinocyte. These cells make up about 95% of the epidermal cell population, the others being melanocytes, Langerhans cells and Merkel cells.

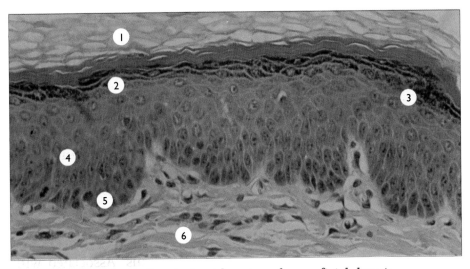

Figure 2.1: Histology of typical epidermis and superficial dermis
1. Stratum dysjunctum; 2. Stratum compactum (these two together form the stratum corneum); 3. Stratum granulosum (granular layer); 4. Stratum spinosum; 5. Stratum basale (basal layer); 6. Stratum (papillary) dermis

Epidermal cells

The keratinocyte is a typical epithelial cell forming the lining of all internal and external body surfaces, eg. mucosal tissues. The epidermis is a stratified epithelium. Keratinocytes begin life from cell division of 'stem' cells at the basement membrane level and in the hair follicle bulge (*Figure 2.3*). They slowly migrate towards the skin surface, differentiating to become first 'spinous' cells, then 'granular' cells (both due to the microscopic appearance), and finally, squames, or stratum corneum cells. These are then lost to the environment in the process of desquamation — this is the orderly loss of cells from the skin surface once their purpose has been served. To illustrate the importance of this process, abnormal desquamation often presents as a disease state, as is the case with ichthyosis vulgaris.

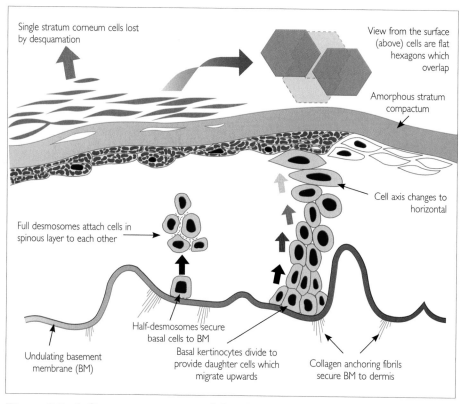

Figure 2.2: A diagrammatic view of the skin section, shown in *Figure 2.1* illustrating key features of epidermal biology

Differentiation is marked by biochemical and morphological changes; each designed to modify the cell for its eventual role in physical protection and permeability barrier function. The newly-formed basal keratinocyte is very much like any other epithelial cell in appearance, but as it differentiates its appearance changes. The spinous cell is so-called because of the histological appearance of its numerous junctions (desmosomes) with neighbouring cells (*Figure 2.2*). These cell junctions affix basal cells firmly to the basement membrane, and, in the layers above, each cell to another. The end result is an epidermis that resists shear forces.

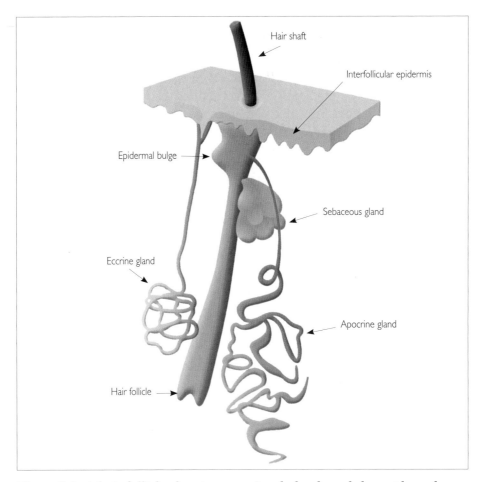

Figure 2.3: A hair follicle showing associated glands and the epidermal stem cell bulge

The production of keratin protein and keratohyaline granules, known as 'keratinisation', within the cell, gives the stratum granulosum cell its characteristic appearance (Matoltsy, 1975). This may be regarded as the last 'living' cell layer in the epidermis as, hereafter, cells enter the stratum corneum where they are little more than flattened sacs of inert protein, devoid of the nucleus and other organelles associated with living cells.

Melanocytes

The pigmentation of human and animal tissues not only provides cosmetic coloration to the skin, hair and eyes, but also gives significant protection to the body from ultraviolet (UV) radiation damage. Failure of this mechanism leads to photoaging and carcinogenesis (eg. melanoma). The melanocyte is the cell most closely associated with the pigmentary system. In the skin, this dendritic cell resides in the basal region of the epidermis, where it synthesises melanin pigment granules (as special organelles — melanosomes) and transfers them to neighbouring keratinocytes. These granules serve to disperse incident UV radiation, so protecting cell nuclei from damage (Hearing, 2005). The distribution of pigment also serves to give the skin and hair its colour (the hair bulb has a melanocyte population). Melanin synthesis is regulated by complex pathways of receptors and hormones (pituitary gland melanocyte-stimulating hormone or MSH: Slominski *et al*, 2004); it is triggered by exposure to UV sunlight and hormones, such as oestrogens and progestogens. In the fetus, by 7-week estimated gestation age, melanocytes are already present in the human epidermis and remain there until hair morphogenesis begins, about two weeks later (Holbrook *et al*, 1989).

Langerhans cells

The skin plays a key role in immune reactions to environmental antigens (see below for more details), and central to that is the Langerhans cell. This is a dendritic cell, derived from bone marrow leucocytes, which resides exclusively in the basal region of the epidermis. These cells, known as 'antigen-presenting' cells, transport antigens from the epidermis to draining lymph nodes (Romani *et al*, 2003). Antigens, such as microorganisms and foreign proteins, are presented to T-helper lymphocytes. In so doing, Langerhans cells regulate processes such as the development of cytotoxic T-lymphocytes, the production of antibodies by B-lymphocytes, and, the activation of macrophages. Langerhans cells therefore play a crucial role in contact sensitisation and in immunosurveillance against viral infections and neoplasms of the skin. These cells are damaged by UV radiation, interfering with their role and where UV exposure is chronic, leading to their depletion. Similarly, the application of potent topical corticosteroids will reduce their numbers.

Merkel cells

At the level of the stratum basale, there is a population of 'neuroendochrine' cells which form a mechanoreceptor function — these are Merkel cells. Evidence shows that cutaneous tactile perception is due, in part, to the complex of Merkel cells and axon terminals of type 1 sensory nerve fibres (Ogawa, 1996; Johnson, 2001; Tachibana and Nawa, 2002). In addition, these cells have been claimed to regulate keratinocyte proliferation and differentiation, but this remains speculative at this time (Tachibana, 1995). In the fetus, Merkel cells are thought to be involved in the induction and alignment of arrector pili muscles (Narisawa *et al*, 1996), formation of eccrine sweat glands (Kim and Holbrook, 1995), and, because of their close proximity to the stem cells, of the bulge (Figure 2.3) paracrine functions (Moll, 1994).

The basement membrane and dermo-epidermal junction

The interface between the epidermis and dermis is defined by a membrane known as the basement membrane. This is made largely from collagens — the important connective tissue proteins (see below) — and provides a secure foundation for the basal keratinocytes, mechanical support for the epidermis, and a semi-permeable filter which regulates the passage of cells and nutrients from dermis to epidermis. The membrane itself is firmly attached to the dermis by means of more collagen-anchoring fibrils. The dermo-epidermal junction (DEJ) develops with age, transforming from a flattened plain in the premature infant, to a deeply ridged zone that makes up rete ridges in infants and children (Hoeger, 2002). The real value of this system of cell anchorage only becomes apparent in disease states where its performance is compromised: thus, in the bullous diseases of pemphigus and pemphigoid, and in epidermolysis bullosa (EB), defective basement membrane function leads to debilitating conditions.

Stratum corneum

The stratum corneum is often regarded as a homogeneous layer; it is, however, two subtly different layers, the lower stratum compactum and the exterior stratum dysjunctum (Bowser and White, 1985). The compactum is the location of the water permeability barrier. Biochemical changes, particularly to lipids, occur as cells metamorphose from 'granular' to 'compactum', providing the barrier property. The stratum dysjunctum is the interface with our environment; the cells here serve as a physical protective material. As they now have no barrier capacity and are porous, they will readily absorb water: the effect we see as reversible maceration. Palmar and plantar skin has a particularly thick stratum corneum, mostly dysjunctum, and is especially prone to maceration (White and Cutting, 2003).

The epidermal permeability barrier

The skin controls moisture vapour loss and protects the individual from the excessive loss which would lead to rapid dehydration. This is measured as transepidermal water loss (TEWL) and is proportional to the site of the body exposed (Yosipovitch *et al*, 2000), the ambient air, humidity, and the gestational age of the infant. Full-term neonates have an average TEWL slightly below that of adults. Thus, TEWL is lower in infants than in adults in the forehead, palms, soles and forearms. Stratum corneum hydration is lower on the forehead, back and abdomen; and higher on palms. The significant anatomic variability in TEWL and hydration should be considered when evaluating the permeation of skin care products and topical medications in the newborn. The younger the infant, the greater the fluid loss. TEWL can be reduced by humidifying the ambient atmosphere (for instance, within an incubator).

Immature epidermis not only allows the passage of moisture into the environment, but can allow the ingress of certain chemicals applied to the skin, including alcohol, urea, antibiotics, such as neomycin, and iodine. Even term infants demonstrate greater absorption of toxic material than adults through the intact skin, but in pre-term infants, absorption is proportional to gestational age, and can lead to neonatal toxicity (Rutter, 1987).

Dryness, whether clinical or sub-clinical, gives the skin a tight, rough feel. While the barrier can keep some chemicals out, its role in this capacity is not absolute. We know that some drugs, for example, corticosteroids and oestrogens, readily penetrate the skin in the context of 'transdermal drug delivery' (Hadgraft, 2004; Prausnitz *et al*, 2004; Thomas and Finnin, 2004).

Vernix caseosa

During the last trimester of fetal development, the baby is covered in a white, fatty, cream-like substance, known as the vernix caseosa. This film is composed of water (80.5%), proteins and lipids (Hoeger *et al*, 2002). It is made in two structures: wax esters are formed in the sebaceous glands while barrier lipids are derived from keratinocytes. It is believed that the vernix forms a barrier to maceration of the developing epidermis from amniotic fluid, and, acts as a host defence. In this respect, vernix contains proteins such as cystatin and calgranulin, which have an antifungal activity, opsonising capacity and protease enzyme inhibition (Tollin *et al*, 2005).

The cutaneous immune system

As the interface with our environment, the skin is the tissue most often confronted with foreign antigens and pathogens (Bos, 1997; Misery, 1997). There are four typical immunological skin reactions: type I includes the immediate hypersensitivity reactions mediated by IgE and mast cells. These include anaphylaxis, angioedema, and wheal flare (histamine release). Type II are the humoral-cytotoxic reactions mediated by complement, IgG and IgM. Type III reactions include vasculitis, and type IV includes granulomatous reactions and delayed hypersensitivity. The dense network of epidermal Langerhans cells (see above) is associated with the skin-specific contact allergy known as delayed hypersensitivity (or type IV reaction). Practitioners in wound care will often see these reactions as allergies to adhesives, dressings, and skin preparations common in patients with venous leg ulceration (Cameron, 2006).

Immune functions of keratinocytes

Epidermal keratinocytes have been recognised as immunocompetent cells and, as such, produce a vast array of immunological molecules (Uchi *et al*, 2000). Keratinocytes are capable of producing interleukins (IL-1α, IL-1β, IL-6, IL-8); colony stimulating factors (IL-3, GM-CSF, G-CSF, M-CST); interferons (IFN-a, IFN-b) tumour necrosis factor (TNF-α); transforming growth factors (TGF-α, TGF-β); and other growth factors (platelet-derived growth factor, fibroblast growth factor) (Bos and Kapsenberg, 1993). Keratinocytes may, therefore, play an active role in the elaboration of molecular signals that facilitate leukocyte homing and local activation, enabling certain dermal cells to mature, and in regulating synthesis of extracellular matrix molecules.

As this is such a complex area, the reader is recommended to consult specialist texts for further details: eg. Roitt IM, Delves PJ *Essential Immunology*, 10th edn, Blackwell Science Publishing London; Baker B (2006) *Skin Immune Mechanisms in Health and Disease*. Garner Press, Beckenham.

The dermis

Underlying the basement membrane zone is the relatively acellular layer known as the dermis. This is a collection of cells and structures that fulfil many of the key functions of the skin, and is predominantly made up of the fibrous proteins, collagen and elastin. These form what is generally known as connective tissue. Suspended in these structures are supportive structures such as the vascular and neurological components. The dermis makes up 15–20% of the total weight of the human body. It varies in thickness from approximately 5mm in areas such as the back and thighs, to as little as 1mm in the skin of the eyelids.

The dermis is regarded as two differing layers with subtle variations in composition, microscopic appearance, and function (*Figure 2.4*). The more superficial papillary dermis is found directly below the basement membrane. It is composed predominantly of a fine woven network of collagen fibres. These run around hair follicles and sebaceous glands, and around eccrine and apocrine glands, as well as between the rete ridges. This region is also rich in hyaluronic acid or hyaluronan. This is a carbohydrate polymer of glucuronic acid, which, in the dermis, forms a viscous gel providing physical cushioning visco-elastic support (Balasz, 2004).

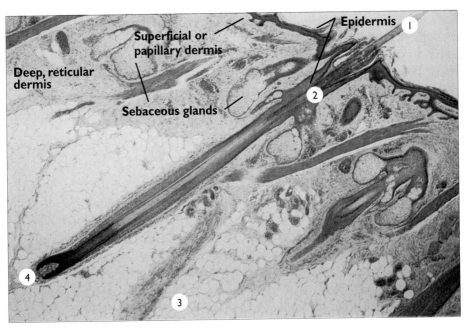

Figure 2.4: This transverse section of human skin shows an area rich in hair shafts and sebaceous glands. Note the scale of the hair, this provides a reference for the thickness of the epidermis. The high density of sebaceous glands is typical of facial or scalp tissues and will result in an oily/greasy skin. Note that the hair follicle is an invagination of the epidermis
1. Hair shaft emerges from the skin surface; 2. Sebaceous glands discharge sebum into the hair follicle; 3. Fat cells in sub-cutis; 4. The hair bulb

The reticular dermis forms the base of the dermal layer and is mainly made up of thicker bundles of collagen fibres.

During life, collagen is continually being broken down and replaced. It is synthesised by cells known as dermal fibroblasts. These cells secrete tropocollagen which, after further extracellular processing, is converted to mature collagen. Normal adult human skin is made up of approximately 85% type I collagen and 15% type III collagen (Gay and Miller, 1978). In fetal life, type III collagen is far more common. These materials provide the skin with its tensile strength.

Elastin fibres are found throughout the dermis. These are also manufactured by the fibroblasts, but their main role is to provide the elastic recoil of the skin. This permits tissues to return to their relative positions after lateral stress, preventing the skin from becoming 'baggy'. Elastic fibres are thicker and more common in the lower levels of the dermis, however, their numbers do not remain constant throughout life. Elastic fibres degenerate with age and exposure to UV radiation. This results in the classic sagging and stretching of the skin we experience in old age.

The gaps between collagen bundles, collagen fibres and elastic fibres are filled with a substance referred to as 'ground substance'. This acts as an amorphous filling agent.

Hair follicles

Hair follicles are first seen during the third month of fetal development. The hair follicle is made up of three areas: the lower section extends from the base of the follicle to the insertion of the erector pili muscle, the middle portion extends from the muscle to the entrance of the sebaceous gland, and the final portion extends from the sebaceous gland to the surface of the skin. The structure of the follicle changes with the growth cycle of the hair. In normal hair development, the active growth phase lasts at least three years, with the regressive phase lasting about three weeks, and the resting period lasting approximately three months. At any one time, about 84% of hair follicles are in the active growth phase (Thiers and Galbraith, 1986).

The hair follicle is lined with epidermal cells and is a downward extension, or invagination, of the epidermis. Although the bulk of this structure is found in the dermis, it should be considered an epidermal component. The 'bulge' area (*Figure 2.3*) is a source of epidermal stem cells and is particularly evident in the fetal lanugo hair (see below: Christiano, 2004; So and Epstein, 2004). In the lower portion of the follicle, cells form the hair matrix from whence the hair itself develops. There are a number of melanocytes found in this area. These are responsible for the production of hair colour. As cells migrate upwards they differentiate and keratinise, the outer layers in each hair hardening first.

Hairs are classified as terminal, vellus, and lanugo. The lanugo hair is first formed _in utero_ on the scalp and face in the second trimester, and all over the body towards the end of that trimester. They are replaced in the child and adult by vellus and terminal hairs (Rogers, 2004).

Sebaceous glands

Sebaceous glands are found in skin throughout the body, except on the palms of the hand and soles of the feet. In most areas they are associated with hair follicles, although in a few areas, notably the areolae, nipples, labia and inner prepuce, they may be found as free structures. Their role is to produce the lipid-rich secretion sebum. These glands are present at birth, but vary in size and action throughout life as a result of hormone stimulation. At birth, sebaceous glands are well-developed and active. This is probably the result of maternal hormone stimulation. Within months, the glands atrophy until puberty, when, under the influence of androgens, glands increase in size and sebum production. At this time they are particularly active in facial skin and in the skin of the nose.

Sweat glands: eccrine, apocrine, and apoeccrine

Eccrine glands primarily serve in the regulation of body temperature through the production of sweat (Sato _et al_, 1989). The gland is formed of a tight coil which lies in the lower third of the dermis, but which may extend down as far as the dermal-subcutaneous fat level. A duct leads from the coil through to a downward projection of the rete ridges, and then finally out onto the surface of the epidermis. The upper portions of this track are lined with epidermal cells, lower structures contain a secretory cell lining. On average, there are 3 million sweat glands in the human skin. These are capable of producing a maximum of 1.8 litres of sweat per hour. This consists of water, salts (predominantly sodium and potassium), as well as numerous proteolytic enzymes indicating that sweat may possess pro-inflammatory or protective functions, as well as being involved in heat regulation.

Apocrine glands are found in distinct areas of the human skin. They are the equivalent of scent glands in humans and are only found in the axillae, in the anogenital region, and as modified glands in the external ear canal, in the eyelid and in the breast (Mizuno *et al*, 2004). Although present at birth, they only begin their secretory action after puberty. We now know that there is a third gland type, the apoeccrine. In the axillae of six-year-old children, both classical apocrine and eccrine glands are present, but no apoeccrine glands were found. Between eight and fourteen years of age, the number of large eccrine glands gradually increases. At 16–18 years of age, the number of apoeccrine glands increases to as high as 45% of the total axillary glands. The data support the notion that apoeccrine glands develop during puberty in the axillae from eccrine or eccrine-like sweat glands (Sato *et al*, 1987).

Blood vessels

The blood vessels of the dermis are divided into two horizontal plains. The superficial vascular plexus is made up of interconnecting arterioles and venules which lie close to the epidermal border and wrap around the structures of the dermis, such as hair follicles. These supply oxygen and nutrients to these rapidly metabolising cells. There is a second network known as the deep vascular plexus. This is found deeper in the dermis at its border to the subcutaneous fat layer. It is made up of more substantial vessels. Vertical vessels connect these two plexus.

The glomus cells are specialised vascular structures that are found in the reticular dermis, mainly in the pads of the fingers and toes, but also in the volar aspect of the hands and feet and in the central facial region. They represent areas of arteriovenous shunting that do not have a capillary network between the arterioles and venules, and are concerned with temperature regulation. When opened, these areas permit the rapid transfer of blood which aids in radiant heat loss.

Mast cells

These cells are part of the immune system. Mast cells are found around blood vessels, nerves and appendages in the dermis, predominantly in the region of the dermal vascular plexus (Eady, 1976). They contain a number of granules. These are extruded from the cell after cross-linking with IgE on the cell surface. Degranulation occurs within minutes of exposure to the stimulant releasing a number of molecules, including histamine. In the skin, this produces relaxation of smooth muscle causing vasodilation. Histamine also increases capillary permeability attracting more leukocytes to the affected area. In time, the mast cells produce inflammatory mediators — prostaglandins and leukotrienes, as well as a variety of cytokines that promote the inflammatory process. In addition, mast cells secrete tumour necrosis factor-α (TNF-α), which acts as a chemo-attractant to neutrophils.

Neural network

It is believed that around 1 million afferent nerve fibres innervate the skin (Sinclair, 1981). The skin is supplied with both sensory and autonomic nerves. The autonomic nerves derive from the sympathetic nervous system and supply the blood vessels, erector pili muscles, eccrine and apocrine glands. Sebaceous glands show an absence of autonomic pathways, relying on endocrine stimulation to activate their function.

Sensory nerves enter the skin at the sub-dermal fatty tissue, each dividing into smaller bundles that fan out in a horizontal plane to form a branching network. These fibres ascend to the superficial dermal layers. Most end in the dermis, however, a number penetrate into the basement membrane. There are a number of different types of sensory receptors in the skin, each one developed to react to one form of external stimuli. The sensations of touch, pressure, heat and cold and pain are mediated by the dendritic endings of different sensory neurons.

The sensation of heat and cold are mediated by simple neurons. The receptors for cold are located in the dermis just below the epidermal junction. They are stimulated by cooling, and inhibited by warming. Receptors for heat are located deeper in the dermis and are fewer in number. Exposure to very high temperatures also produces the sensation of pain. This occurs as a result of the activation of a particular protein — a capsaicin receptor. High temperatures, or exposure to capsaicin, the chemical in chilli peppers which causes the 'burn' results in ion channels being opened. This permits the diffusion of Ca^{2+} and Na^+ ions into the neuron producing depolarisation.

This ultimately stimulates the central nervous system, permitting the perception of heat and pain.

Pain is also perceived through action of specialist pain receptors. These naked receptors transmit electrical activity through the axon to the spinal cord, where they synapse, and the stimuli is transmitted to the higher centres of the brain. Sharp pain sensations are transmitted through myelinated axons, capable of transmitting impulses rapidly; whereas dull pain and ache is transmitted via slower non-myelinated axons. There is evidence that ATP released from damaged cells, along with a local fall in pH (for instance, following inflammation and infection), also stimulate these receptors, leading to pain.

Touch sensations, so important to the neonate (Anderson *et al*, 2003), are mediated through simple nerve endings surrounding hair follicles, and specialist nerve endings called Merkel's discs and Ruffini endings. Touch and pressure are also mediated by dendrites encapsulated within various structures, including Meissner's corpuscles and pacinian corpuscles. These structures are found in the dermis throughout the individual, but are most heavily concentrated in the hands and feet, particularly in the finger tips.

Muscle cells

The dermis contains a number of muscle fibres. Smooth, involuntary muscle makes up the erector pili apparatus which is responsible for elevating body hair — producing goose-bumps, but is also found in the nipple. Striated muscle is found in the neck (platysma) and in the face where it controls fine facial movement and facial expression.

Lymphatic system

In normal conditions the skin has a rich lymphatic system. This is responsible for the transportation of particulate and liquid material, such as protein from the extravascular compartment of the dermis. Broad lumen vessels with single cell thick walls transport fluid away from the skin, and to the lymph nodes maintaining homeostasis in the tissues.

Skin functions

Temperature regulation

In evolutionary terms, the development of warm-blooded animals had a significant impact on the animal world and the evolution of the mammals. Through the maintenance of a relatively constant core temperature, it was possible to maintain rapid cell metabolism regardless of climatic conditions. This, however, does have a major problem; the need to preserve heat and dissipate excess heat energy as the need arose.

Heat regulation in the developing fetus provides a number of challenges to physiological function. Being warm blooded, humans maintain a core temperature within a narrow operating range. _In utero_, the fetus has a higher metabolic rate than the mother and so the fetal temperature is generally 0.3°C to 0.5°C higher than an adult, (Power, 1989). Eighty-five percent of heat energy produced by the fetus is passed to the mother via the placental interface. The remaining 15% is dissipated into the amniotic fluid and is transferred to the maternal abdomen. The reduction of blood flow through the umbilical cord can result in fetal core temperature rising. This can occur during delivery. This theory is supported by Asakura's research (1996), which demonstrated higher skin temperatures immediately post-delivery in babies which had suffered umbilical cord coiling.

Immediately following birth, the baby faces a hostile environment, where the ambient temperature is considerably lower than that experienced _in utero_. It is essential that the baby generates heat to compensate for the lost energy. This is achieved through shivering and non-shivering thermogenesis (NST). The shivering response in newborn infants is immature as skeletal musculature is poorly developed; it is therefore an insignificant coping mechanism. What is apparent, is the role of non-shivering thermogenesis. Brown adipose tissue, found in full-term infants is rich in mitochondria, has a well-established sympathetic nerve system, and has a rich blood supply. It is able to generate heat energy and utilise this to raise core temperature. It is believed that this response is stimulated by the relatively high post-delivery oxygen levels in the infants circulation, and the absence of chemical inhibitors derived from the mother or the placenta

(Takeuchi *et al*, 1994; Ball *et al*, 1995). NST has been demonstrated to be closely associated with neonatal oxygenation with a strong correlation between umbilical pO_2 and NST activity (Asakura, 2004).

Brown adipose tissue is laid down in the developing fetus in the latter stages of pregnancy, infants delivered pre-term may have compromised thermogenesis potential. In Asakura's study, infants delivered prior to 30 weeks gestation did not exhibit NST activity. In addition, these infants had thinner skin layers, making them more prone to heat loss.

Neonates have much higher numbers of sweat glands than adults; however, sweating to achieve maintenance of core temperature is far less pronounced (Mancini and Lane, 1998). The intensity of the sweating response depends on the gestational age. Premature infants are normally unable to sweat for the first few days of life, unlike full-term infants, however, sweating in response to chemical stimuli can be initiated in infants as young as 32 weeks gestation.

The ability to sweat is established in all infants soon after birth, and is prompted in pre-term babies by environmental factors. By day 13, even premature infants display sweating to thermal stimuli, even if less effectively than their full-term counterparts.

The greatest threat to neonates is heat loss, which is normally achieved by evaporative loss rather than radiant exchange within the first few weeks of independent life. Infants do not demonstrate the same ability to constrict surface blood vessels to conserve heat that is seen in older children.

In the child, the neural network of the skin provides an accurate measure of ambient temperature through the activation of heat and cold receptors in the dermis. Signals are passed via the nerve pathways to the hypothalamus, which can initiate the inhibition of sweating or the initiation of shivering. Ambient stimuli have little influence on core body temperature, other than getting us to reach for that extra layer of clothing — it therefore has more of a behavioural influence than a physiological one.

What does have a significant effect is the major role the skin plays in direct thermoregulation in the child, and subsequently, the adult. Excess heat can be lost through the skin by conduction, convection, radiation and evaporation. Sweating, a function of the eccrine glands, permits the dissipation of excess heat energy by evaporation, while the dilatation and constriction of the rich blood vessels in the dermal plexus enables heat energy to be modified in the underlying structures. Damage to this skin function, through burns or inflammatory conditions, such as severe eczema and Stevens-Johnson syndrome, can lead to catastrophic collapse and is often referred to as 'skin failure' (Irvine, 1991).

Vitamin D synthesis

The production of 1,25-dihydroxyvitamin D_3 begins in the skin, where vitamin D_3 is produced from its precursor molecule under the influence of sunlight. Vitamin D_3 is an essential component in calcium regulation in the body, and so affects bone deposition and serum calcium levels. It has also been postulated that it acts as an autocrine regulator of the epidermis. This idea is supported by the action of UV light and vitamin D analogues on the skin in patients suffering from psoriasis, where it inhibits cell proliferation and promotes differentiation of keratinocytes (Fox, 2002).

Protection against ultraviolet radiation

As well as visible light, the sun produces a range of radiation that is invisible to the naked eye, but which has an effect on the function of the skin. UV light is made up of two main wave bands. The shorter wavelength, UVB rays, are able to penetrate the epidermis and cause sunburn and, in the long term, skin cancer. Longer wavelength, UVA rays, are believed to be the major cause of skin changes associated with ageing.

The skin has two methods of protection against UV radiation; a pigmentation barrier formed by melanin, and a protein barrier found in the stratum corneum. Both act by minimising the absorption of harmful radiation by cellular DNA, therefore minimising the genetic mutation potential.

Communication

In many ways, the skin can be viewed as a 'window to the soul'. Owing to the influence that systemic disease can have on the appearance of the skin, whether through colour, texture, temperature or function, clinicians can use it as an indicator of inner body functions and well-being of the individual — as a way of assessing general health and diagnosing disease. As such, clinicians need to be able to recognise normal and abnormal cutaneous phenomena that present themselves — they need to learn to read the signs.

Outside the purely medical context, while it may appear obvious, the skin is the one structure that we see when we communicate with other humans. In particular, facial movement and expression is used as a method of communicating mood, emotion, and as a primary method of identification, particularly in the mother-infant relationship (Mizuno *et al*, 2004). The ability to influence sensation through touch is used as a primary method of expressing bonding (Anderson *et al*, 2003), and can even be an analgesic for the infant (Gray *et al*, 2000). From the moment of birth, changes in the function or appearance of the skin can have profound effects on how we perceive those around us, and ourselves.

References

Anderson GC, Moore E, Hepworth J *et al* (2003) Early skin-to-skin contact for mothers and their healthy newborn infants. *Cochrane Database Syst Rev* **2**: CD003519

Asakura H (1996) Thermogenesis in fetus and neonate. *J Nippon Med School* **63**: 171–2

Asakura H (2004) Fetal and neonatal thermoregulation. *J Nippon Med School* **71**: 360–70

Balasz EA (2004) The viscoelastic properties of hyaluronan and its therapeutic use. In: Garg H, Hales C, eds. *Chemistry and Biology of Hyaluronan.* Elsevier publications, London: chap 20

Ball KT, Takauchi M, Power GG (1995) Role of prostaglandins I^2 and E^2 in the initiation of non-shivering thermogenesis during the simulation of birth in utero. *Reprod Fertil Dev* **7**: 65–119

Bos JD (1997) The skin as an organ of immunity. *Clin Exp Immunol* **107**: suppl 1: 3–5

Bos JD, Kapsenberg ML (1993) The skin immune system: progress in cutaneous biology. *Immunol Today* **14**(2): 75–8

Bowser PA, White RJ (1985) Isolation, barrier properties, and lipid analysis of stratum compactum, a discrete region of the stratum corneum. *Br J Dermatol* 112: 1–14

Christiano AM (2004) Epithelial stem cells: stepping out of their niche. *Cell* 118(5): 530–2

Eady RAJ (1976) The mast cells: distribution and morphology. *Clin Exp Dermatol* 1: 313–21

Fox C, Nelson D, Wareham J (1998) The timing of skin acidification in very low birth weight infants. *J Perinatology* 18: 155–9

Fox SI (2002) Regulation of metabolism. In: Vander A, Sherman J, Luciano D, eds. *Human Physiology*. 7th edn. McGraw Hill, London: 607

Gay S, Miller S (1978) *Collagen in the Physiology and Pathology of Connective Tissue*. Gustav Fischer Verlag, Stuttgart

Gray L, Watt L, Blass EM (2000) Skin-to-skin contact is analgesic in healthy newborns. *Pediatrics* 105(1): 14

Hadgraft J (2004) Skin deep. *Eur J Pharm Biopharm* 58(2): 291–9

Hearing VJ (2005) Biogenesis of pigment granules: a sensitive way to regulate melanocyte function. *J Dermatol Sci* 37(1): 3–14

Hoeger PH, Schreiner V, Klaassen IA *et al* (2002) Epidermal barrier lipids in human vernix caseosa. Corresponding ceramide patterns in vernix and fetal epidermis. *Br J Dermatol* 146: 194–201

Hoeger PH, Enzmann CC (2002) Skin physiology of the neonate and yound infant. Prospective study of functional skin perameters during early infancy. *Pediatr Dermatol* 19: 256–62

Holbrook KA, Underwood RA, Vogel AM, Gown AM, Kimball H (1989) The appearance, density and distribution of melanocytes in human embryonic and fetal skin revealed by the anti-melanoma monoclonal antibody, HMB-45. *Anat Embryol* 180: 443–55

Irvine C (1991) 'Skin failure' — a real entity: discussion paper. *J Roy Soc Med* 84: 412–13

Johnson KO (2001) The roles and functions of cutaneous mechanoreceptors. *Curr Opin Neurobiol* 11(4): 455–61

Kim DK, Holbrook KA (1995) The appearance, density, and distribution of Merkel cells in human embryonic and fetal skin. *J Invest Dermatol* 104(3): 411–16

Madison KC (2003) Barrier function of the skin: 'la raison d'etre' of the epidermis. *J Invest Dermatol* 121(2): 231–42

Mancini AJ, Lane AT (1998) Sweating in the neonate. In: Polin RA, Fox WW, eds. *Textbook of Fetal and Neonatal Physiology*. 2nd edn. WB Saunders, Philadelphia: 767–70

Matoltsy AG (1975) Desmosomes, filaments, and keratohyaline granules: their role in the stabilisation and keratinization of the epidermis. *J Invest Dermatol* **65**(1): 127–42

Misery L (1997) Skin, immunity and the nervous system. *Br J Dermatol* **137**(6): 843–50

Mizuno K, Mizuno N *et al* (2004) Mother-infant skin-to-skin contact after delivery. *Acta Paediatr* **93**(12): 1640–5

Moll I (1994) Merkel cell distribution in human hair follicles of the fetal and adult scalp. *Cell Tissue Res* **277**(1): 131–8

Narisawa Y, Hashimoto K, Kohda H (1996) Merkel cells participate in the induction and alignment of epidermal ends of arrector pili muscles of human fetal skin. *Br J Dermatol* **134**(3): 494–8

Ogawa H (1996) The Merkel cell as a possible mechanoreceptor cell. *Prog Neurobiol* **49**(4): 317–34

Power GG, (1989) Biology of temperature: the mammalian fetus. *J Dev Physiol* **12**: 295–304

Prausnitz MR, Mitragotri S, Langer R (2004) Current status and future potential of transdermal drug delivery. *Nat Rev Drug Discov* **3**(2): 115–24

Rogers G E (2004). Hair follicle differentiation and regulation. *Int J Dev Biol* **48**: 163–70

Romani N, Holzmann S, Tripp CH *et al* (2003) Langerhans cells — dendritic cells of the epidermis. *APMIS* **111**(7/8): 725–40

Rutter N (1987) Percutaneous drug absorption in the newborn: hazards and uses. *Clin Perinatol* **14**: 911–30

Sato K, Kang WH, Saga K, Sato KT (1989) Biology of sweat glands and their disorders. I. Normal sweat gland function. *J Am Acad Dermatol* **20**(4): 537–63

Sato K, Leidal R, Sato F (1987) Morphology and development of an apoeccrine gland in human axillae. *Am J Physiol* **252**(1 part 2): R166–80

Sinclair DC (1981) *Mechanisms of Cutaneous Sensation*. 2nd edn. Oxford University Press, Oxford

Slominski A, Tobin DJ *et al* (2004) Melanin pigmentation in mammalian skin and its hormonal regulation. *Physiol Rev* **84**(4): 1155–228

So PL, Epstein EH (2004) Adult stem cells: capturing youth from a bulge? *Trends Biotechnol* **22**(10): 493–6

Tachibana T (1995) The Merkel cell: recent findings and unresolved problems. *Arch Histol Cytol* **58**(4): 379–96

Tachibana T, Nawa T (2002) Recent progress in studies on Merkel cell biology. *Anat Sci Int* **77**(1): 26–33

Takeuchi M, Yoneyama Y, Power GG (1994) Role of prostaglandin E^2 and prostacyclin in nonshivering thermogenesis during simulated birth in utero. *Prost Leukotr Essential Acids* **51**: 373–80

Thiers BH Galbraith GMP, (1986) Alopaecia areata. In: Thiers BH, Dobson RL, eds. *Pathogenesis of Skin Diseases*. Churchill Livingstone, New York: 57

Thomas BJ, Finnin BC (2004) The transdermal revolution. *Drug Discov Today* **15**(9): 697–703

Tollin M, Bergsson G, Kai-Larsen Y *et al* (2005) Vernix caseosa as a multi-component defence system based on polypeptides, lipids and their interactions. *Cell Mol Life Sci* **62**(19): 2390–9

Uchi H, Terao H, Koga T *et al* (2000) Cytokines and chemokines of the epidermis. *J Derm Sci* 24(Suppl 1): S29–S38

Yosipovitch G, Maayan-Metzger A, Merlob P, Sirota L (2000) Skin barrier properties in different body areas in neonates. *Pediatrics* **106**(1 Pt 1); 105–8

Chapter 3

Principles of neonatal skin care

Valerie Irving

Skin care for the neonate varies depending on the gestation at birth and the postnatal age. Pre-term infants born before 33 weeks gestation, when the skin becomes functionally mature, encounter different problems from those born at term.

The main aim of any skin care protocol should be to maintain the integrity of the skin. An initial skin assessment should be carried out at, or as soon as possible after birth, so that a base line can be documented and any abnormalities recorded. Thereafter, assessments should be updated on at least a daily basis, or more frequently for the very pre-term infant, ie. 6–8-hourly, or as their condition changes.

Evidence-based guidelines should direct staff to appropriate cleansing regimes; which products to use and which to avoid. The provision of a supportive environment is essential to maintaining skin integrity, using soft sheeting and positioning aids to reduce the potential for the infant to suffer friction injuries from irritability. Careful repositioning will help reduce pressure or ischaemic injuries, but must be considered along with the infant's general condition so that deterioration is not caused by this intervention.

At any gestation, products which are applied to the skin should not have the potential to cause more harm than good, and should be assessed according to need and their appropriateness for that individual infant.

Should any injury occur, it must be treated using the most effective evidence-based treatment, with careful documentation to monitor rates of healing.

Term/post-term infant

At term, the skin is similar in structure and function to that of an adult (Rudy, 1991). The subcutaneous fat is usually well developed; however, the dermis is odematous with small collagen bundles and immature elastin fibres. The epidermis is composed of cuboidal cells which divide and differentiate from the stratum basale into the stratum spinosum, the stratum granulosum and, finally, the stratum corneum (*Chapter 2*). Throughout the process, the cells become flattened as the nuclei die, and are filled with keratin, which gives the skin its waterproofing barrier layer (Butcher and White, 2005). This layer is responsible for protecting the body from chemicals, bacteria, heat and light, as well as regulating water loss through the skin. Although the epidermal layers are thinner than those of an adult, they are well developed. However, there is still potential for the percutaneous absorption of any products applied topically, as the infant has a large skin surface to weight ratio. If the child is born after 42 weeks gestation, the nails are keratinised and may be long, curved and stained green, due to the passage of meconium *in utero* caused by increasing placental insufficiency (Rudy, 1991). Nails should be kept short so that infants cannot scratch their skin, but care must be taken not to damage the nail bed, which will bleed and be a site for infection (Lin *et al*, 2004).

Temperature control is limited, even at term, as, due to their immature eccrine glands, infants cannot lose heat by sweating until two to three weeks of age. The first bath should only be given when the infant's temperature has stabilised, as allowing the infant to become cold will increase oxygen requirements. The ingredients of any commercial products used in bathing and skin care should be evaluated before use, as many contain perfumes and dyes which are irritant and drying to the skin. Within the first month of life, the average neonate can be exposed to up to 66 different chemicals from these type of products alone, all of which have the potential to be absorbed (Cetta, 1991).

Washing

The development of the acid mantle, the body's bactericidal property, begins at birth, when the pH of the skin is initially 6.34. If born at term, the process of pH reduction to below 5 takes three to four days; for the premature infant this process can take several weeks (Lund *et al*, 1999).

Unless specifically identified as having an acid pH (ie. below 7), soap-based products tend to be alkaline with a pH of up to 9. These alter the skin's pH after use, increasing it above the pH 5 optimum. It can take up to one hour for the skin of the term infant to regain its acid property; for the premature infant, this takes even longer, thus interfering with its protective acid mantle. This allows proliferation of bacterial growth and increases the permeability of the skin surface (Gfatter *et al*, 1997).

In many cases, plain water is adequate for washing. If soap solutions are thought to be necessary, once or twice a week is sufficient (da Cunha and Procianoy, 2005) and, even then, the product should be rinsed off before drying the infant.

da Cunha and Procianoy (2005) found that the act of bathing, using either mild pH-neutral soap products or plain water, reduced the number of colony-forming units of both Gram-positive and Gram-negative bacteria found on the skin, but did not influence the type of organisms.

Using antimicrobial products for bathing

The use of antimicrobial products has been found to be unnecessary, as their effect on skin flora are only transient. Caution is urged in using hexachlorophene (HCP) for routine bathing, as past history has shown that it causes infant death from neurotoxicity (West *et al*, 1981).

At birth, the skin of a post-term infant tends to be wrinkled and looks macerated. By a few hours after birth, it takes on a paper-like appearance and begins to peel and crack. The use of emollients or moisturisers may be beneficial for these infants, but there is the potential for skin irritation, an allergic reaction, or toxicity to occur through percutaneous absorption.

Moisturisers add water to the stratum corneum and have a limited effect, while emollients enhance the epidermal hydration by repairing the barrier function, and restoring the diffusion of water from the dermis to the epidermis (Horii and Lane, 2001).

Emollients can be in ointment, cream, or lotion form. Ointments, which are more greasy, consisting of soft paraffin, or a combination of soft, liquid and hard paraffin, are more occlusive and are, therefore, usually more effective (British National Formulary [BNF], 2003).

Care of the umbilical cord stump

This varies in practice: the most common being the use of antiseptic agents such as alcohol, silver sulfadiazine, iodine, chlorhexidine, or triple dye (brilliant green, proflavine hemisulphate and crystal violet in aqueous solution). Some authorities recommend the use of antibiotics, and others just to keep it clean and dry (Zupan _et al_, 2005). Following a review of 21 studies by the Cochrane Collaboration, antiseptic use was shown to delay the time to separation of the cord, but reduced maternal concern about the cord. However, Zupan _et al_ (2005) concluded that the limited research did not show any advantage in the use of antibiotics or antiseptics over just keeping the cord clean and dry.

Nappy rash

This is a type of contact dermatitis, which is only found in the nappy area and is caused by contact with faeces or urine (_Chapter_ 7). Although the most common age to develop nappy rash is nine to twelve months, it can be found in the term and pre-term population. It was often thought to be the ammonia in the urine which caused the nappy rash, however, this is now known to be incorrect (Borkowski, 2004). The prolonged contact with a urine-soaked nappy can lead to maceration of the stratum corneum, and this becomes more susceptible to damage from the enzymes or proteases found in faeces.

There is an increased incidence of a rash when the infant has suffered diarrhoea, been receiving antibiotics, or recovering from neonatal abstinence syndrome, as the increased movement of faecal matter through the gastrointestinal tract increases the activity of the proteases (Atherton, 2004).

The use of alcohol- and perfume-free cleansing wipes is not recommended in the pre-term infant.

Barrier products

Clinical evaluations of commercially available barrier products should provide the evidence base on which to choose the most effective product. However, there are not sufficient studies carried out, and products are often chosen by the strength of the marketing rather than established therapeutic value (Atherton, 2004). The ideal product works by adding a lipid layer to the surface of the skin, and/or providing lipids which can penetrate the stratum corneum, simulating the effects of naturally occurring lipids. These will protect the skin from irritants and microorganisms and prevent increased transepidermal water loss through any damaged areas (Atherton, 2004). Some barrier products work by containing water-repellent substances, but there is no evidence that they are any more effective than traditional ones.

Lambe (2001) commented that, previously, it had been thought that too great an application of a barrier product, such as white soft paraffin, would act as an occlusive product and prevent any recovery to the damaged area. However, Lambe (2001) said that petrolatum permeates through the stratum corneum interstices, allowing normal barrier recovery despite its occlusive properties. There has been little research into the effectiveness of the many available products, some of which contain unnecessary antibacterial/antifungal components (Borkowski, 2004). Sudocrem® (Tosara Products UK) is one such product, which has a fungistatic action against *Candida albicans* by preventing the growth of spores (Allison, 2000) while Drapolene® (Warner Lambert) contains cetrimide, an effective antiseptic.

Where nappy rash is severe, a paste is the product of choice as it has a thick consistency and adheres to the broken moist area, eg. Granuflex paste® (ConvaTec) or Orabase® (ConvaTec). These products do not have to be removed at each nappy change, thus preventing further damage to the healing skin.

Nappy rash caused by infection from *Candida albicans* presents in a different manner, and may occur alone or with oral thrush. The area is covered with bright red papules, erythematous plaques, and pustules with characteristic satellite lesions along sharp borders. Treatment with topical antifungal ointment should be applied several times a day. Nystatin® (Squibb) acts by binding to the sterols in the fungal cell membrane, thereby losing both its barrier function and cell constituents. Treatment should continue until the swabs taken for culture are clear on two occasions. Oral antifungal therapy should commence at the same time, and continue for the same period, to prevent re-infection from any spores contained in the gastrointestinal tract.

For resistant candida infections, imidazole agents, such as clotrimazole and miconazole, should be considered (Lambe, 2001).

At 36–38 weeks gestation, the skin may be covered with a white sebaceous material called vernix caseosa. This protects the skin from maceration while *in utero*, and is gradually shed over the first few days of life. There is no need to try and remove this for cosmetic reasons, as it is felt to have some bactericidal and waterproofing property protecting the skin (Haubrich, 2003).

Survival at 23–24 weeks gestation is in the region of 50%, and the problems of immature skin cause much concern to the staff providing intensive care. As no subcutaneous fat has developed at this stage, the skin has a red appearance and the dermis, which is in direct contact with the muscle layer, is oedmatous, leaving the skin gelatinous to the touch.

Transepidermal water loss

At 23–24 weeks gestation the stratum corneum has not yet developed, therefore, there is no barrier function for the skin, resulting in a high transepidermal water loss of up to 110 mls/kg/day (Harpin and Rutter, 1983). If fluid intake is not carefully monitored, this can lead to imbalance and dehydration. Modern, double-walled incubators, which are able to maintain an effective humidified environment of up to 90% (relative humidity, RH). At this RH, transepidermal water loss is reduced to virtually nil, and the effects of evaporation, conduction, convection and radiation are prevented. While nursed in this environment, the infant should not be dressed as the clothes become damp; plastic sheeting is unnecessary, as this interferes with the circulation of the warm moist air. The canopy should not be allowed to mist up, as this indicates that the environmental temperature is having a cooling effect, even through the double walls, and droplets of the cool moisture can fall onto the infant. A humidified environment should be maintained for two to three weeks, with humidity levels being reduced over this period to 40% before being discontinued. Studies by Harpin and Rutter (1985) found that the skin rapidly matures once the environment of a fluid-filled uterus is exchanged for a gaseous one, and, after a 2–3-week period, the skin should act similarly to that of a term infant without excessive transepidermal water loss.

The use of radiant heaters gives the carers and parents better access to the infant, however, the direct heat source increases the potential for transepidermal water loss and, although humidified air can be pumped into an improvised plastic tent, it is not as effective as that found in an electronically regulated, humidified, double-walled incubator. Also, it cannot be monitored, and increases the risk of scald injuries occurring.

Transepidermal water loss can be reduced by applying emollients to the skin. Rutter and Hull (1981) showed that a mixture of 80% soft paraffin and 20% hard paraffin could reduce the levels by up to 60% and, more recently, Nopper *et al* (1996) used Aquaphor® (Smith & Nephew) twice daily, and found a reduction of 67% just 30 minutes after application. This product is not available in the UK. Consideration must be given for the potential of any product applied to the skin to be absorbed and become toxic. For example, in the 1970s, a commonly used skin cleansing preparation, hexachlorophene, was used in liquid form which resulted in raised blood levels of the compound. Accidental contamination of talcum powder with concentrated hexachlorophene caused infant deaths and, postmortems of the most vulnerable infants who died, showed intermyelin oedema and vacuolation. Consequently, the product was removed from neonatal use (West *et al*, 1981) .

Chemical burns

Alcohol-based solutions should only be used with caution, washed off using sterile water, and any soaked material replaced prior to the procedure commencing, to prevent unnecessary prolonged contact. Harpin and Rutter (1982) reported serious burns on the backs of infants from the use of alcohol-based cleansing solutions which had soaked into sheeting and had not been removed before the procedures were carried out. The danger of alcohol use was supported by a report from Watkins and Keogh (1992), who described similar injuries due to the use of alcohol-impregnated wipes in a neonatal unit in Australia. Isopropyl alcohol can be absorbed through the skin of the premature infant, resulting in raised blood alcohol levels; studies in adults have found residual Gram-negative and -positive organisms after its use (Choudhuri *et al*, 1990).

Linder *et al* (1997) described how the use of iodine-based cleansing solutions caused transient hypothyroidism when used on pre-term infants. Aqueous chlorhexidine has the least toxic or damaging effects on pre-term skin when compared to iodine- or alcohol-based solutions.

Although it does have the potential to be absorbed through the skin of the pre-term infant, this does not appear to have any detrimental effect (Rutter, 1987). Chlorhexidine is effective against a wide range of bacteria, yeasts and some fungi, and its use is widespread in neonatal units as part of skin preparation prior to invasive procedures (Siegfried, 2001).

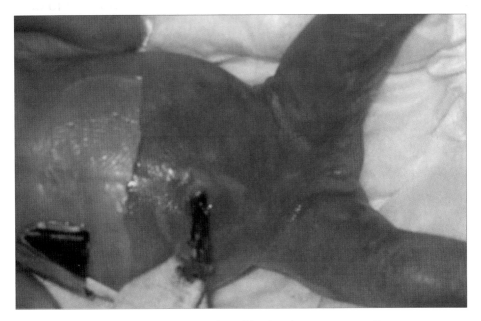

Figure 3.1: Chemical burn. Reproduced by kind permission of Fiona Burton

Heat burns

Although a rare occurrence, heat burns can occur from the use of fibre optic 'cold lights' used to illuminate blood vessels prior to cannulation. It is important that the use of these are time-limited, and any covers or guards are used appropriately.

Epidermal stripping

The skin of the pre-term infant is susceptible to epidermal stripping, as the fibrils which anchor the epidermis to the dermis are few in number and more widely spaced than in more mature skin. Epidermal stripping occurs when the bond between any adhesive product used and the surface of the epidermis is stronger than that between the epidermis and the dermis, so that on removal of the adherent product, epidermal layers are stripped off with it. This includes the use of all adhesive monitoring products and tapes used to secure catheters, drains and tubes.

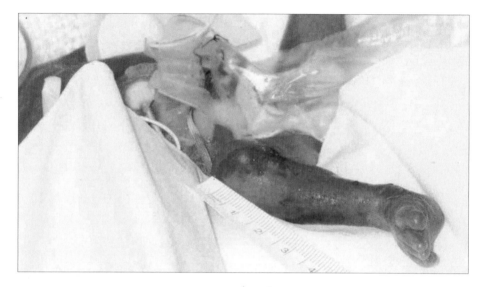

Figure 3.2: Epidermal stripping

To reduce damage, a hydrocolloid base layer (Duoderm®, ConvaTec) can be used on the skin to attach tape and other adhesive products to it. This product can stay in place even if the tape is removed for repositioning or removal of the catheters etc, and be removed at a later date when no longer required.

Neither the use of bonding agents, nor solvent removers, are appropriate in this group of patients, as they increase the risk of skin damage and toxicity due to percutaneous absorption. Tape can be double-backed to prevent contact, or rubbed with cotton wool to reduce its adhesive properties.

Pressure/ischaemic injuries

As discussed before, the dermis is oedematous at birth. This can put pressure on the tiny blood vessels which lead to the epidermis, making it more prone to pressure damage.

Due to the large surface area to weight ratio, injuries which do occur are rarely found in what are considered to be the typical pressure areas. However, infants who are unstable, requiring inotropes for hypotension, paralysing agents, or are sedated for ventilation, are more at risk, with the ears and the occiput being the most common sites of damage.

With each set of nursing care procedures, the position of the ears should be checked to prevent unnecessary pressure on them. The hat used to secure oral endotracheal tubes should also be checked to ensure good positioning and that it has not become too tight; this would cause undue pressure around the edges and under the ties. Careful positioning regimes and the use of supportive boundaries will reduce the risk of such injuries occurring by preventing the infant from becoming fractious and unsettled.

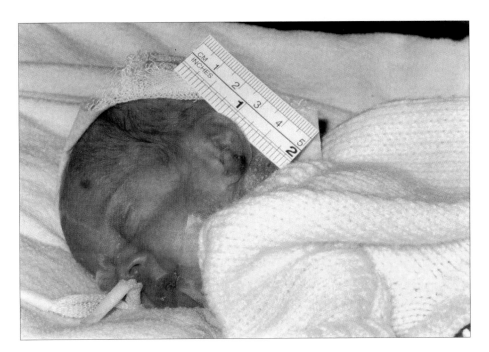

Figure 3.3: Pressure/ischaemic injury

Monitoring devices, such as saturation probes, can cause pressure/ischaemic injuries. Depending on the gestation and general condition of the infant, these should be repositioned frequently to prevent indentation of the skin and pressure damage occurring.

By continually improving antenatal care, high risk pregnancies are being prolonged longer than was previously possible, and infants are being born with skin injuries noted at delivery. These can be due to pressure from the uterine walls when the amniotic fluid has leaked, from the cord or other body parts, or even from amniotic bands which have ruptured. It is important both to document such injuries carefully, and to take photographs to determine the causative factors and rule out the possibility of any iatrogenic involvement.

Extravasation injuries

To compare British figures assessing the significance of rates of extravasation injuries with those from the USA is difficult as definitions are different. British studies clearly differentiate between failed infusions which do not cause tissue damage, and those which do. Infiltration of fluids is said to occur when there is non-intentional leakage of a non-vesicant fluid which resolves without damage. Extravasation occurs when there is the non-intentional leakage of a vesicant fluid into the tissues, leading to cell and tissue death.

Extravasation injuries are by far the most serious injuries which can occur, and the resulting scarring is a life-long reminder of the incident. A recent survey of regional intensive care units found a prevalence of 38 per 1 000 neonates sustaining an injury which resulted in skin necrosis. Most injuries occurred in infants of 26 weeks gestation or less, who had parenteral nutrition infused through peripheral cannula (Wilkins and Emmerson, 2004).

Such injuries can occur when irritant fluids, for example, total parenteral nutrition (TPN), dextrose greater than 10%, and some drugs which are hypotonic and/or have a high pH, are given intravenously rather than by central lines. Any irritation of the blood vessel walls can lead to a chemical phlebitis, causing back-flow of the solution through the cannula site and into the surrounding tissue. The tip of the cannula can become dislodged and puncture the wall of the vessel with similar results. Hecker *et al* (1991) found that the median life span of peripheral intravenous infusion sites was 36 hours, with TPN infusions lasting for shorter periods than dextrose infusions.

Should central lines not be a viable option for any infant due to size, infection, instability, or the inability of clinical staff to insert the line, then careful siting of any cannula is essential. A record of the cannulation must be kept, including the site used, number of attempts taken, the name and designation of the person who performed the cannulation, the condition of the skin and surrounding area, as well as the size and type of cannula used.

Once in place, the cannula should be secured with a sterile, clear film dressing which allows continual visibility of the site. Nursing programmes must ensure that it is checked at least hourly for signs of displacement, leakage, swelling, blanching, or redness. A record of these checks must be kept, with the person responsible noting any action required, who this was carried out by, and when.

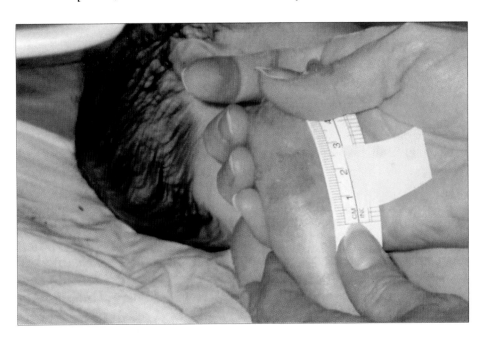

Figure 3.4: Extravasation injury

There is no nationally recognised assessment tool for checking cannula sites in the neonatal population, with many units adapting adult tools such as the one devised by Jackson (1998).

Any change in the colour or condition of the area requires further investigation, and the cannula may need to be removed.

Film dressings themselves, if used on the very pre-term infant, have the potential to cause epidermal stripping on removal. However, an evaluation of a non-alcoholic barrier film spray used on the skin beneath these dressings showed a reduction in the number of such injuries (Irving, 2001).

Splints used to support the limb can be secured with Velcro® straps, but these must not occlude any visibility of the site and area around the tip of the cannula. On a very active infant, Velcro® straps are not effective and may need to be replaced with clear tape which has been double-backed, or had the adhesive backing reduced with cotton wool to prevent epidermal stripping injuries occurring.

Skin assessment tools

Skin assessment tools have not been accepted on a national basis, although many units use their own locally devised tool, which reflects the gestation and acuity of the infants they care for, but is not research-based.

Due to the lack of suitable alternatives, tools have been based on pressure sore prediction tools for adults (*Chapter 5, pp. 79–86*). Even paediatric tools, such as the Waterlow paediatric risk assessment tool (1997), was found to be unsuitable for the very young infant (Waterlow, 1997).

One specific tool for neonates is the 'Neonatal Skin Risk Assessment Scale' (Huffines and Logsdon, 1997). However, this score groups all the infants below 28 weeks gestation into one group, and one of the factors includes the use of a saran tent under a radiant heater which is not used in the UK.

More recently, Lund *et al* (2001) devised the 'Neonatal Skin Condition Score', which records three factors of dryness, erythema and skin breakdown on a twice-weekly basis. The mean gestation of infants used to devise this tool was 33 weeks and, again, it is not appropriate for those of a much lower gestation.

A useful tool should include a range of assessments which are non-subjective and easily recorded on a frequent basis. It should cover a wide range of gestations, and not exclude those born nearer to term, despite the fact that the challenges of maintaining skin integrity are greatest for the lowest gestations. It should suggest strategies to be used to prevent any injuries becoming worse, as well as appropriate wound contact products.

Lund *et al* (2001) reported on the improvement in skin assessment and care following a large multi-centred study involving specific teaching of neonatal staff, and the development of guidelines. This study, involving nearly 3000 infants, covered 51 neonatal units in North America, and resulted in many positive changes in practice.

Although many units follow evidence-based practice in this country, similar work is required with collaboration between those in neonatal, paediatric and adult tissue viability areas, together with product manufacturers, to produce national guidelines and teaching packages which could be disseminated to all units, regardless of the number or acuity of infants.

References

Allison F (2000) Nappy rash: an overview. *Practice Nurs* **11**(17): 17–19

Atherton D (2004) A review of the pathophysiology, prevention and treatment of irritant diaper dermatitis. *Curr Med Res Opin* **20**(5): 645–9

Borkowski S (2004) Diaper rash care and management. *Pediatr Nurs* **30**(6): 467–70

British National Formulary (2003) Royal Pharmaceutical Society of Great Britain. British Medical Association, London

Butcher M, White R (2005) The structure and functions of the skin. In: White R, ed. *Skin Care in Wound Management: Assessment, prevention and treatment*. Wounds UK, Aberdeen

Cetta F, Lambert G, Ros S (1991) Newborn chemical exposure from over–the–counter skin care products. *Clin Pediatr* **30**: 286–9. Cited in: Malloy-McDonald M (1995) Skin care for high risk neonates. *J WOCN* **22**: 177–82

Choudhuri M, Mc Queen R, Inoue S, Gordon R (1990) Efficiency of skin sterilization for a venipuncture with the use of commercially available alcohol or iodine pads. *Am J Infect Control* **18**: 82–5

da Cunha M, Procianoy R (2005) Effect of bathing on skin flora of preterm newborns. *J Perinatol* **25**(6): 375–9

Gfatter R, Hackl P, Braun F (1997) Effects of soap and detergents on skin surface pH, stratum corneum hydration and fat content in infants. *Dermatology* **195**: 258–62

Harpin V, Rutter N (1983) Barrier properties of the newborn infants skin. *J Pediatr* **102**: 419–25

Harpin V, Rutter N (1985) Humidification of incubators. *Arch Dis Child* **60**: 210–24

Harpin V, Rutter N (1992) Percutaneous alcohol absorption and skin necrosis in a pre-term infant. *Arch Dis Child* **57**: 477–9

Haubrich KA (2003) Role of the vernix caseosa in the neonate. *AACN Clin Issues* **14**(4): 457–64

Hecker J, Duffy B, Fong T, Wyer M, (1991) Failure of intravenous infusions in neonates. *J Paediatr/Child Health* **27**: 175–9

Horii K, Lane A (2001) Evidence-based use of emollients in neonates. *Newborn Infant Rev* **1**(1): 21–4

Huffines B, Logsdon C (1997) The neonatal skin risk assessment scale for predicting skin breakdown in neonates. *Issues Comprehensive Pediatr Nurs* **20**: 103–14

Irving V (2001) Reducing the risk of epidermal stripping in the neonatal population: an evaluation of an alcohol free barrier film. *J Neonatal Nurs* **7**(1): 5–8

Jackson A (1998) A battle in vein: infusion phlebitis. *Nurs Times* **94**(4): 68–71

Lambe M (2001) Topical agents in infants. *Newborn Infant Rev* **1**(1): 25–34

Lin R, Tinkle L, Janniger C (2004) Skin care of the healthy newborn. *Cutis* **75**: 25–30

Linder N, Davidovitch N, Reichman B (1997) Topical iodine-containing antiseptics and sub-clinical hypothyroidism in pre-term infants. *J Pediatr* **131**: 434–9

Lund C, Lane A, Raines D (1999) Neonatal skin care: the scientific basis for practice. *JOGNN* **28**: 241–54

Lund C, Osborne J, Kuller J et al (2001) Neonatal skin care: clinical outcomes of the AWHONN/NANN evidence-based clinical practice guideline. *J Gynaecol Neonatal Nurs* **30**: 41–51

Nopper A, Kimberly A Sookdeo-Drost S et al (1996) Topical ointment therapy benefits premature infants. *J Pediatr* **128**: 660–9

Rudy S (1991) From conception to birth: the development of skin and nursing care implications. *Dermatol Nurs* **3**(6): 381–90

Rutter N, Hull D (1981) Effects of applying topical agents. *Arch Dis Child* **56**: 673–5

Rutter N (1987) Drug absorption through the skin: a mixed blessing. *Arch Dis Child* **62**: 220–1

Siegfried E (2001) Neonatal skin care and toxicology. In: Eichenfield LF, Friedon IJ, Esterley NB, eds. *Textbook of Neonatal Dermatology*. WB Saunders, Philadelphia

Waterlow J (1997) Pressure sore risk assessment in children. _Paediatr Nurs_ **9**(6): 21–4

Watkins A, Keogh E (1992) Alcohol burns in the neonate. _J Paediatr Child Health_ **28**: 306–8

West D, Worobec S, Solomon L (1981) Pharmacology and toxicology of infant skin. _J Investigative Dermatol_ **76**: 147–50

Wilkins C, Emmerson A (2004) Extravasation injuries on regional neonatal units. _Arch Dis Child Fetal Ed_ **89**: F274–5

Zupan J, Garner P, Omari A (2005) _Topical Umbilical Cord Care at Birth_ (Review). Cochrane Library Issue 3, John Wiley & Sons Ltd, Chichester

CHAPTER 4

PRINCIPLES OF PAEDIATRIC WOUND MANAGEMENT

Trudie Young

The principles of paediatric wound management should follow those laid down in 'Getting the right start: National Service Framework (NSF) for Children, standard for hospital services' (Department of Health [DoH], 2003). The NSF focuses on services in hospitals to ensure that the care delivered is genuinely child-centred. It provides a template for services designed specifically for children which incorporate the child's point of view. It acknowledges that child-friendly services are different from those provided for adults. It states that child-centred hospital services are services that:

- consider the whole child, not simply the illness being treated
- treat children as children, and young people as young people
- are concerned with the overall experience for the child and the family
- treat children, young people and parents as partners in care
- integrate and co-ordinate services around the child's and family's particular needs
- graduate smoothly into adult services at the right time
- work in partnership with children, young people, and parents to plan and shape services and to develop the workforce.

Although written for hospital care, it emphasises the need for child-centred integrated care across different disciplines and care settings. This reflects current care delivery in which over 80% of all episodes of illness in children are managed by parents without reference to the professional healthcare system. The points at which children usually access the healthcare system are via doctors' surgeries, accident and emergency departments, outpatient clinics, hospital wards, including intensive care units and special care baby units (DoH, 2003). In all settings, healthcare professionals should build pathways of care around the child and the family which results in flexible, responsive and integrated care.

Child-centred paediatric wound management

The developmental age periods for children are illustrated in *Figure 4.1*. However, it is important to remember that the child's chronological age may not match the anticipated developmental age. Therefore, the clinician should not presume a certain level of developmental maturity within the child. It is important that care is designed around the child's developmental age, rather than their chronological age. Children's mental capacity and level of understanding, for example, about their bodies, illness and wounds, may differ from that of most adults, and may change as they develop. In essence, the actual age is less important than the needs and preferences of the individual child.

The goals of holistic wound management in children are to alleviate pain, lessen emotional distress, and minimise scarring (Bale and Jones, 2006). However, it must be remembered that when we nurse children we are nursing the family (Casey, 1999). If the tissue viability team is to integrate and co-ordinate services around the child's and family's particular needs, they will need to act as part of the wider team caring for the child, rather than as a specialist and individualised unit. A small, but increasing number of disabled children with complex health requirements, are now surviving into adulthood (DoH, 2003). There is the likelihood that this client group will have tissue viability concerns. The tissue viability team needs to ensure that they support these children during their appropriate integration into adult services.

Prenatal period:	conception to birth
Germinal conception to approximately 2 weeks	
Embryonic:	2–8 weeks
Fetal:	8–40 weeks
Infancy period:	birth to 12 months
Neonatal:	birth to less than 28 days
Infancy:	1–approximately 12 months
Early childhood:	1–6 years
Toddler:	1–3 years
Preschool:	3–6 years
Middle childhood:	6–11 years
Late childhood:	11–19 years
Adolescence:	13–approximately 18 years
	(beginning at the onset of puberty and ending at adulthood)

Figure 4.1: Developmental age periods. Adapted from Whaley and Wong, 1999

Safety within paediatric wound management

The NSF states that hospitals should be safe and healthy places for children. For example, in accident and emergency and minor injury departments, surgery recovery areas and outpatient clinics there should be a physical separation between child and adult patients. This is to ensure that children are not exposed to potentially frightening scenes and behaviours, and equally, that adults who are feeling ill are not disturbed by noisy children (DoH, 2003). Children associate events, people and places with unpleasant or painful experiences, which can have lasting consequences (Casey, 1999). The potential of specialist units and teams to overlook the safety of the child was highlighted by the report into children's heart surgery at the Bristol Royal Infirmary chaired by Professor Ian Kennedy ('The Kennedy Report') (Bristol Royal Infirmary Inquiry, 2001). It found hospitals operating in self-contained worlds, as if the prior experience of the child in front of them had no bearing, and as if what happened to them afterwards, or outside the hospital, was of no concern. It is imperative that the tissue viability team consider the safety and the wider picture of the child when in their care.

Within a hospital setting, the child's bed space is viewed as a place of safety and their own sanctuary. Therefore, unless unavoidable, any wound-related procedures should be carried out in areas other than the bed space. Treatment and dressing rooms can be a frightening environment for a child, filled with scary looking equipment, metal trolleys and instruments, and large glaring overhead lights. Nevertheless, this can be altered and improved to make them child-friendly areas. The door to the room can be made welcoming and the equipment draped in brightly coloured fabric. Once in the room, the focus can be adapted to the needs of the child and include mobiles, television and DVD screens. Audio input can also enhance the environment. Ceiling lights and hoists can be converted into spaceships, and natural distractions, such as fish tanks, can provide relaxing visual distractions (*Figure 4.2*).

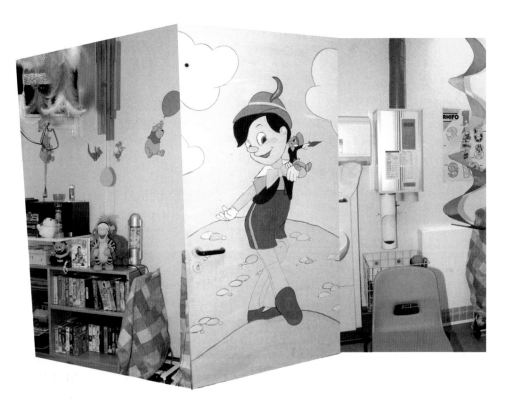

Figure 4.2: Paediatric treatment rooms. Reproduced by kind permission of Glan Clwyd paediatric outpatients and Mike Jones, hospital photographer

Pressure-relieving equipment should be suitable for the length and weight of the child. If this is not acknowledged, the weight of the child may not be distributed evenly across the support surface and the child may find limbs slipping between the cells. Some products require body heat and weight to facilitate the spreading of the load across the support surface. This may be problematic during infancy. There exists equipment that has been designed specifically for children, such as the Nimbus® paediatric range (Huntleigh Healthcare Limited).

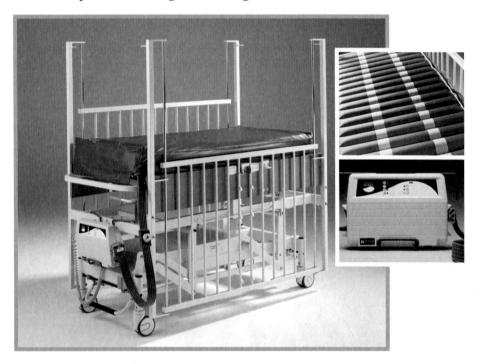

Figure 4.3: Nimbus® paediatric pressure-relieving equipment. Reproduced by kind permission of Huntleigh Healthcare Limited

The wound management plan for a child should be, at best, evidence-based, and, if this is not possible, evidence-linked. The latter may often be the benchmark due to the paucity of clinical trials of wound management products that involve children. Where the evidence does exist, it should be utilised, eg. tissue adhesives to close simple facial lacerations (Osmond, 2000).

It is important to consider the physical repair capabilities of the child. In general, children have a greater capacity for healing; however, they often lack the reserves to counteract significant systemic events (Garvin, 1990). The tissue viability team should be watchful and attentive when dealing with children who are at risk of developing wound infection. In children, signs of systemic infection can vary from those of an adult, and include fever, restlessness, and general malaise.

Vigilance should also be part of the wound assessment process in situations where a non-accidental injury is suspected. Regrettably, it may be necessary to restrain a child during certain procedures. During periods of restraint, and when dealing with children who have suffered a non-accidental injury, the tissue viability team should be aware of the national and local guidance on restraint and child protection.

Protection of the child may extend to dressing retention methods, for example, a full-hand bandage may be necessary to secure a dressing in a child who is prone to place their hand in their mouth (Independent Multidisciplinary Advisory Group [Tendra Academy], 2004). The mobility and activity levels of the child can increase the risk of dressing dislodgement, which can have serious consequences; child-friendly dressings can help secure intravenous cannulae (McCann, 2003). Factitious injuries are known to occur in young people. An audit of a general paediatric ward, over an eight-month period, identified that fifty-eight children between the ages of 11 and 17 had been admitted following a deliberate act of self-harm (Marfe, 2003). The tissue viability team will need to assist the young person during these times of crisis and refer to other healthcare professionals for additional support.

Respect and choice in paediatric wound management

The views of the child and family should be paramount in paediatric wound management. The general principle is founded within the United Nations Convention for the Rights of the Child, article 12 (17), 'children have a right to be involved in decisions about their care'. A respectful partnership with a child's parents ensures that the tissue viability team recognises that the parents are usually the experts on their child (DoH, 2003). An example of where this failed to happen was highlighted in The Kennedy Report (2001), when children's rights were overlooked and there was an absence of an open and honest relationship between healthcare professionals, children, and their parents as partners in care.

Real choices over aspects of treatment or care should be offered to the child wherever possible. For a younger child, this could include choice about where to sit during a procedure, the colour of the dressing, and whether it is opaque or transparent, and if they wish to look at the wound during the procedure. Nevertheless, it should be remembered that most products are developed for adults and have not been tested in small children, and often the size of dressing hampers its use in babies (Van Riet and Van Dam, 2003). Children should be involved in choices between wound management options, or about who should deliver the wound care. The Department of Health (2004) suggest that, wherever practicable, young people should be offered choice regarding the gender of the professional they see. Choices made about wound care should be recorded in the nursing care plan. Play techniques can help children and young people understand the options and exercise choice (DoH, 2003). Encouraging parents and children to take responsibility for their wound management where appropriate, prepares for discharge home and allows the tissue viability team to assess the child's and parents' abilities to cope with complex wound management therapies, eg. topical negative pressure therapy (TNP) (Butter *et al*, 2006). Children need to be tempted to eat to improve their healing potential. They should be able to decide what they want to eat; unfamiliar or strange foods should be avoided, and choices for children and families should acknowledge their cultural needs (DoH, 2003). Children and parents can take responsibility for other factors affecting the healing process, ie. curtailing activities if necessary, assessing the condition of the wound, redressing, and seeking advice if they have concerns. This may extend to long-term regimens, eg. massage and pressure garments to improve the cosmetic appearance of scarring (Casey, 1999). The various stages of empowerment should be considered to allow for choice in participation, that is within the child's and family's abilities. This may be a dynamic process, with responsibility being increased and relinquished at various stages of the healing process (Independent Multidisciplinary Advisory Group [Tendra Academy], 2005).

Children's best interests are served, on the whole, by being in hospital for the briefest possible time needed to provide safe and effective treatment. Evidence also suggests that most parents would prefer to care for their sick child at home, where this is an option (DoH, 3003). Hospital is disruptive to the child and family and to the care of other children; it can be costly to the family in terms of travel, parking, meals at the hospital, time off work and extra child care for siblings. Parents' time is valuable and they may need to take time off work to accompany their child to hospital appointments, and repeated visits might mean they lose pay. In addition, parents may have their own health or other problems to deal with; and this may affect their understanding of explanations offered, and their readiness to participate in the treatment of their child. Health care can impose material hardship, for instance, when a child is in hospital a long way from home. Parents may have other children to care for, and will have to balance their needs with the needs of the child in hospital (DoH, 2003). The tissue viability team will need to consider the above, rather than, as is often the case, what is the optimum environment for wound management. They should also bear in mind the pressure of the situation, where a parent has to display their parenting skills in a public arena. In addition, the parent may feel guilty regarding the cause of the wound and have anxieties about managing the wound. This may affect their ability to participate in care. The tissue viability team should allow the child and the parent to develop their skills at their own pace, with privacy and dignity.

Communication

Children and parents can only participate fully as partners in care if they have access to accurate information that is valid, relevant, up-to-date, timely, understandable and developmentally, ethically and culturally appropriate (DoH, 2003). Communication should also help to convey practical issues, eg. a child may find an epithelialising wound itchy, the risk of keloid scarring in children with pigmented skin, and which dressings contain animal products.

A range of communication methods should be developed and used, and information should be available about specific conditions, procedures, services and support groups, in a variety of formats, media and languages, eg. burned children's club (Independent Multidisciplinary Advisory Group [Tendra Academy], 2004). Audio or video tapes of the most common procedures carried out in the paediatric unit are helpful. In addition, audio recordings of consultations have been suggested as a means of improving communication with children and their families. There is some evidence that adult patients and parents value this approach, and that it improves information recall and satisfaction (DoH, 2003). Clinicians might consider offering audio recording of consultations to improve communication in certain circumstances, perhaps where complex and difficult information is being shared: for example, with families of children with cancer or babies in neonatal intensive care.

The sharing of information is important. However, parents with disabled children report some frustrating issues, ie. healthcare professionals who do not know the child insist on taking the child's details again; parents get fed up with having to tell the same painful story over and over. The solution is a good summary in the notes, with a copy held by the parents, so that staff can concentrate on the acute episode that has brought the child into hospital.

The NSF (DoH, 2003) suggests that play may be used for therapeutic purposes, ie. as a way of helping the child to:

- assimilate new information
- adjust to and gain control over a potentially frightening environment
- prepare to cope with procedures and interventions.

Depending on the child's age, understanding, and perception of the wound, its cause and meaning for the future will vary widely and will change over time (Casey, 1999). The child's description of the wound may not match that of the healthcare professional, and the child may use different language for body areas. If it is the child's first experience of a wound, they will lack the history and life experience that would help them communicate with the tissue viability team. However, it is imperative that the healthcare professional establishes the child's understanding, fears, experiences, and feelings about the wound. Rogers (2003) asked healthcare professionals, parents and children to help them elicit meaningful terms to describe skin lesions, focusing on distribution, shape, size, colour and texture. Examples of terms they suggested include nasty, sore, horrible, lumpy, bumpy, scabby (rice crispies). They caution against using items for comparisons that come in a variety of sizes, eg. buttons, and suggest using comparisons with known items of fixed size, eg. coins. Preparing the child for wound dressing changes is an important part and one in which parents can be invaluable, eg. rocking, cuddling and trust are ways that pain and distress can be reduced in infants (Melhuish and Payne, 2006). Distraction techniques are helpful to reduce distress in both younger and older children. Wood (2002) developed a leaflet about distraction to help empower parents during painful procedures.

Communication should be a two-way event, and the tissue viability team should obtain feedback from children and parents as to the quality of the service they provide. This will ensure that the views of children and parents are heard, and their opinions and suggestions used to develop the service. The Department of Health (2004) recommend using 'tell us what you think forms' to elicit feedback from children.

Table 4.1: Types of wounds seen in children	
Infants	
Surgery:	appendectomy, circumcision
Accidents:	burns, scalds, head injuries and dog bites
Excoriation:	due to nappy rash or dribbling
Chronic disorders:	haemangioma, epidermolysis bullosa
Non-accidental injuries	
Congenital abnormalities:	homozygous protein C deficiency (Benbow and Pearce, 1994)
Extravasation injuries	
Early childhood	
Surgery:	appendectomy, circumcision
Accidents:	burns, scalds, hand injuries, dog bites, abrasions and broken limbs — falling off bikes
Pressure ulcers in children with physical/learning disabilities	
Middle childhood	
Accidents:	road traffic injuries, burns from fireworks, lacerations
External fixation trauma following broken limbs	
Leg ulcers:	sickle cell disease
Late childhood	
Factitious injuries	
Infection:	meningoccocal septicaemia
Intervention-related injuries:	extravasation
Surgery:	pilonidal sinus

Adapted from the Independent Multidisciplinary Advisory Group, 2004

Conclusion

The principles of child-centred care, respect and choice, safety and communication should underpin paediatric wound management. The tissue viability team will need to recognise their limitations and that, for once, the parent rather than themselves may be the expert. They should take the lead from others, for example, the ability of a children's nurse to help and show parents rather than completing the task on their behalf. The standard set by the Department of Health (2004) applies to paediatric wound care in that:

> *Children and young people and families should receive high quality services which are co-ordinated around their individual and family needs and take account of their views.*

References

Bale S, Jones V (2006) *Wound Care Nursing. A patient-centred approach.* 2nd edn. Elsevier Ltd, London

Benbow M, Pearce C (1994) The care of an infant with homozygous protein C deficiency. *J Wound Care* 3(1): 21–4

Bristol Royal Infirmary Inquiry (2001) Learning from Bristol: the Report of the Public Inquiry into Children's Heart Surgery at the Bristol Royal Infirmary 1984–1995. Cm 5207. July. Stationery Office, London. Available online at: www.bristol-inquiry.org.uk

Butter A, Emran M, Al-Jazaeri A, Ouimet A (2006) Vacuum-assisted closure for wound management in the pediatric population. *J Pediatr Surg* 41(5): 940–2

Casey G (1999) wound management in children. *Paediatr Nurs* 11(5): 39–44

Department of Health (2003) *Getting the right start: National Service Framework for Children, standard for hospital services.* Stationery office, London

Department of Health (2004) *Every Child Matters: Change for Children in Health Services.* Stationery Office, London

Garvin G (1990) Wound healing in pediatrics. *Nurs Clin North Am* 25(1): 181–92

Independent Multidisciplinary Advisory Group (2004) *Issues in paediatric wound care minimising trauma and pain.* Tendra Academy, Mölnlycke Health Care

Independent Multidisciplinary Advisory Group (2005) *Issues in Wound Care: Communicating with and Empowering Patients. Report from An Independent Advisory Board.* Tendra Academy, Mölnlycke Health Care

Kumar KA, Kumar E (1993) A pressure sore in an infant. *J Wound Care* 2(3): 145–6

Marfe E (2003) Assessing risk following deliberate self-harm. *Paediatr Nurs* 15(8): 32–4

McCann B (2003) Securing peripheral cannulae: evaluation of a new dressing. *Paediatr Nurs* 15(5): 23–6

Melhuish S, Payne H (2006) Nurses' attitudes to pain management during routine venepuncture in young children. *Paediatr Nurs* 18(2): 20–3

Osmond MH (2000) Wound repair and tissue adhesives. In: Moyer VA *et al*, eds. *Evidence-based Pediatrics and Child Health.* BMJ Books, London

Rogers D (2003) Skin assessment: improving communication and recording. *Paediatr Nurs* 15(10): 20–3

Van Riet JM, Van Dam A (2003) Pressure ulcers in children. *European Pressure Ulcer Advisory Panel Review* 5(1): 24, 25

Wood C (2002) Introducing a protocol for procedural pain. *Paediatr Nurs* 14(8): 30–3

Wong D, Hockenberry M, Wilson D, Winkelstein M, Ahmann E, DiVito-Thomas P (1999) *Whaley & Wong's Nursing Care of Infants and Children.* Mosby, St Louis

Chapter 5

Pressure ulcer risk assessment in children

Jane Willock

A pressure ulcer has been defined as:

Damage to the skin caused by pressure, shearing forces or friction, or a combination of these.

(Dealey, 1991)

There are thought to be three main forms of mechanical force acting on body tissues that can cause pressure ulcers: compression, shear and tension. Compression is a force exerted perpendicularly over a given area when underlying tissues are directly compressed, and greater pressures result in greater damage. The duration of pressure is as important as the intensity, and short periods of high pressure, such as sitting on a bedpan, can be as damaging as prolonged periods of lower pressure. Interface pressures are transmitted through all internal tissues (Gould, 2001) and can lead to an area of deep ischaemia. Shear is the force exerted parallel or at an angle to skin surface, causing layers of tissues to move laterally producing severe distortion. This happens especially when patients slide down the bed or are pulled up the bed and the skin moves against the bed sheets; the resulting shearing forces stretch and squeeze the very small vessels leading to capillary, venule and lymphatic disruption. This leads to an area of skin with inadequate blood supply, tissue ischaemia and necrosis. Friction tends to occur when the skin has been allowed to rub against another surface, for example, when elbows or heels rub against bed clothes the epidermis is stripped away to create shallow blisters; this is usually superficial but very painful. Tissue impairment arising from shear force or friction could be avoided with correct patient handling techniques, positioning and equipment (Gould, 2001). Skin tension has a similar effect to shear and can be seen when sticky adhesive tape is used. When the tape is removed, it pulls on the skin causing blistering (Davis, 1998).

A pressure ulcer risk assessment is a model which can be used to predict which patients are at risk of developing pressure ulcers, and which patients are not at risk. Screening tests like this are useful where there is an important health problem that can be improved by early detection using a simple reliable valid tool; but risk assessment scales were only designed to assist, not replace, clinical judgement (Watkinson, 1996). One of the major reasons for using risk assessment scores is because they offer a rapid and convenient way of identifying patients at risk, and their degree of risk. Although experienced nurses can identify high-risk patients, a risk assessment scale can focus attention, and it is also a useful guide for inexperienced nurses. However, they are only useful as part of a complete risk-based programme. Using a scale without knowledge, skill, time and equipment will not have the desired effect (Halfens, 2000).

Good standards of care help to identify and prevent pressure ulcers, but patients may not be monitored closely if they are not considered to be in an 'at-risk' category — especially if circumstances change quickly. The incidence of pressure ulcers will only fall if patients are assessed and reassessed (Gould, 2001).

Risk assessment scales can be used to support clinical decisions and provide objective comparisons of dependency between different departments (Maylor and Roberts, 1999).

How are risk assessments developed

The first published pressure ulcer risk assessment scale, the Norton scale, originated from a survey of elderly people. Pressure ulcer risk assessment tools were initially developed by identifying factors believed to predispose people to pressure ulcers, and combining them into risk assessment tools. These tools were formulated according to the insights of experts at the time they were developed. The individual predictive value of each item was not considered, nor was a comprehensive analysis of all variables performed (Haalboom *et al*, 1999). Many studies into pressure ulcer risk are retrospective (Edwards, 1996a) and, therefore, do not have the qualities of randomisation and control that would be expected from studies with a sound methodology. As the scales in current use do not appear to have been constructed or validated using rigorous statistical methods, their use as risk calculators may be unreliable (Deeks, 1996).

Paediatric pressure ulcer risk assessment tools

Of eight published paediatric risk assessment tools identified (Bedi, 1993; Garvin, 1997; Huffines and Logsdon, 1997; Pickersgill, 1997; Cockett, 1998; Olding and Patterson, 1998; Waterlow, 1998; Loman, 2000), only one (Waterlow 1998) did not have a numerical scoring system. Full details of seven paediatric risk assessment scales are given at the end of the chapter (*pp. 79–86*).

Bedi's (1993) risk assessment was developed in paediatric intensive and high care units. Cockett (1998) developed pressure ulcer risk assessment for children in intensive care based on literature. Garvin (1997) published a 'Patient assessment tool for assessing patients at risk for development of pressure-related breakdown', but does not state how the tool was developed. The Braden Q pressure ulcer risk assessment tool for children is a modified adult scale (Loman, 2000). The risk score was based on the clinical judgement of expert nurses who assessed children. Reliability and predictive validity have been tested for the Braden score with adults, but there does not appear to be any published data for the reliability or validity of the Braden Q with children. Huffines and Logsdon (1997) adapted the Braden scale for use with neonates. Sensitivity was reported to be 83% and specificity was 81% (the published article does not give details of risk scoring). Pickersgill (1997) describes a paediatric pressure ulcer risk assessment which was devised by combining Medley and Waterlow risk assessments. The paediatric tissue viability policy at Pickersgill's Trust (Derbyshire Children's Hospital) included the lifting and handling policy, as incorrect movement of patients could cause shear and friction leading to tissue breakdown. The Pattold pressure scoring system (Olding and Patterson, 1998) was devised for critically ill children by identifying the components necessary for the maintenance of good skin integrity, then listing what the authors considered to be the eight key areas. Each of the eight areas were given a score of 1 to 3; when these were totalled the child could be assigned as low, medium or high risk. Waterlow's (1998) paediatric pressure ulcer risk assessment was developed using the data obtained in her incidence study (Waterlow, 1997). This risk assessment does not involve a numerical score, but alerts users to potential risks and advises on preventative action.

Although the Braden Q scale (Loman, 2000) includes a category for friction/shear, only two risk assessments (Cockett, 1998; Waterlow, 1998) actually mention pressure injury caused by equipment, even though there is published evidence implicating equipment in the development of pressure ulcers. In Groeneveld *et al's* (2004) prevalence study, the most frequent sites for pressure ulcers in children were the ears (33%), which could be attributed to nasal cannulae. 27.3% of pressure ulcers in children in Waterlow's (1997) survey appeared to be associated with equipment. Curley *et al* (2003), Samaniego (2003), and Willock (2005) also reported a significant proportion of children with pressure ulcers attributable to objects or equipment pressing or rubbing on the child's skin. In these situations, a single number obtained from a numerical score will not give any indication of the action needed to prevent pressure ulceration.

The risk assessment tools give similar risk weightings to most characteristics, so a child who is mobile, but has nutrition, elimination, or other problems, could theoretically have a higher risk score than an immobile child.

Reliability and validity

Two properties of a measuring instrument are fundamental — reliability and validity. Unlike a child's temperature, height or weight, their pressure ulcer risk cannot be measured directly. It must be measured by assessing several individual factors that have been implicated in the development of pressure ulcers. Reliability is the extent to which an instrument yields the same results on repeated trials. Inter-rater reliability refers to the variance in scores when a number of raters assess the same patient (Watkinson, 1996). If two or more people weigh a child on the same scales in the same conditions in a short space of time, they would expect to observe the same weight, as this is an objective measure. But a pressure ulcer risk assessment tool measures several conditions, and some of these (such as nutritional status and sensory perception) are subjective, so if two independent people assess the child, there is less chance that they will get exactly the same score. To reduce subjectivity, the meaning of the different criteria should be unequivocal (MacDonald, 1995). It is unlikely that patients will be assessed by the same nurse every time their condition is evaluated, so a risk assessment tool should be as objective as possible to make it reliable, no matter who is doing the assessment (MacDonald, 1995).

A measuring scale is valid if it measures what it was designed to measure. For example, if the weight of a child is being recorded and the child is weighed fully clothed, then the weight of the child and the child's clothes will be measured. This will not be an accurate measure of the child's weight and is, therefore, not valid. If a scale designed to measure pressure ulcer risk actually measures the general health of the patient rather than the risk of developing a pressure ulcer, it is not a valid tool for measuring pressure ulcer risk.

Risk assessment tools are constructed from subscales, each of which assesses a different facet of risk. Risk may be due to any individual factor or a combination of factors; therefore, it may be more important to look at individual risk factors than at overall risk score, such as considering alternative positioning to reduce shear and friction (Deeks, 1996). Potential harm could occur if decisions about interventions were made on the basis of a single score which inappropriately summarises something which has a multifaceted nature (Deeks, 1996).

An assessment tool must contain all relevant items; this is called content validity. In pressure ulcer risk assessment, the assessment tool must be made up of several measurable, observable indicators, such as mobility, activity and nutritional status (Halfens, 2000). There may be over 100 contributing factors which could influence the development of pressure ulcers, either alone, or in combination (Halfens, 2000), however, it would not be practical to incorporate all of these into an instrument. For a scale to be easy to use in practice it should have 10 items at the most. Another problem is how to assess or weigh the risk each item poses (predictive validity), so that the test will give a good prediction of the outcome. Many scales amalgamate the scores from each item in the risk assessment to give a cumulative score. A cut-off point is used to differentiate high-risk patients from low-risk patients, but it is necessary to know where the cut-off point should be, and one point may differentiate between risk categories (Halfens, 2000).

Sensitivity and specificity

As mentioned above, pressure ulcer risk assessment scales that amalgamate scores from individual items such as mobility and nutrition, give a total risk score. This score may give an indication as to whether a patient has a high or a low risk of developing a pressure ulcer. Sensitivity and specificity together indicate the validity of a tool. Sensitivity is the degree to which the tool accurately identifies all persons who are at risk of developing the condition (pressure ulcer); specificity is the degree to which the test will identify all persons who are not at risk of developing the condition (pressure ulcer). These are difficult to assess as the **risk** of developing a pressure ulcer is not the same as **actually** developing a pressure ulcer. All risk scores will appear to be performing poorly if preventative care is effective — good nursing care should prevent the predictions of pressure ulcer development from coming true (Deeks, 1996). If a patient declared 'at risk' does not develop a sore it does not mean that the risk did not exist (Waterlow, 1995). A patient who is immobile and may be at risk of developing a pressure ulcer may not do so because nurses and other healthcare workers reposition him or her frequently enough to prevent damage occurring. To determine true sensitivity and specificity would mean withholding preventative intervention and allowing tissue breakdown in vulnerable patients, which would be ethically unacceptable (Flanagan, 1995).

Studies of predictive validity are limited, in that they assess only the potential that risk assessments possess in separating individuals into 'at risk' and 'not at risk' groups.

Tests need to have a high sensitivity to identify correctly patients with the condition. They also need a high specificity to identify which patients are not at risk and, therefore, will not develop the condition. The implications of a risk score can be substantial, in that an increased risk of developing a pressure ulcer according to the score may imply the use of expensive equipment and intensive nursing input (Haalboom *et al*, 1999).

A high specificity is needed so that resources will not be wasted on patients who will not develop pressure ulcers regardless of level of preventative care; a scale which hugely over-predicts will not be acted on (Edwards, 1996b).

For risk assessment tools to be useful in preventing pressure ulcers, there must be effective interventions available that will prevent patients from developing pressure ulcers, and the use of the risk assessment tool must lead to more appropriate and faster use of resources in patients who will benefit, than would have happened if the risk assessment tool had not been used. The greatest use of risk assessment tools may be their use in developing pressure ulcer prevention protocols which combine assessments of risk factors with recommendations for care and further surveillance. Risk assessment tools may not help nurses to identify all relevant risk factors (Deeks, 1996). If it is not possible to remedy or reduce risk factors, there may be a need to use pressure-reducing equipment.

Receiver–operator characteristics

A receiver–operator characteristics (ROC) curve is a plot of the true positive rate (sensitivity) against the false positive rate (1 – specificity) for given score weightings or thresholds (Anthony *et al*, 2003). The area under the curve is calculated and can indicate whether any randomly selected patient at risk of developing a pressure ulcer will have a higher score than any patient not at risk of getting a pressure ulcer (Anthony, 1996). The larger the area under the ROC curve is, the more effective the scale is at predicting risk.

Conclusion

Pressure ulcers are injury to the skin and underlying tissues caused by pressure, shearing forces and/or friction. A pressure ulcer risk assessment is a model which can be used to predict which patients are at risk of developing pressure ulcers, so that preventative intervention can be taken. They are generally composed of several subscales, such as mobility, nutrition and skin condition, and generally amalgamate risk scores from individual items to give an overall risk score. To be useful, a risk assessment tool must measure what it is designed to measure, it must be reliable, and it must identify patients at risk and patients who are not at risk. The validity of a risk assessment tool can be estimated from patient data using sensitivity and specificity calculations, and the area under the receiver–operator characteristics curve.

Most published pressure ulcer risk assessment tools for infants and children are modified adult scales, or were developed using experiential and anecdotal data. All except the Waterlow paediatric risk assessment tool have a numerical scoring system. There is little information on the reliability or validity of these scales.

References

Anthony D, Reynolds T, Russell L (2003) A regression analysis of the Waterlow score in pressure ulcer risk assessment. _Clin Rehabilitation_ 17(2): 216–23

Anthony D (1996) Receiver operating characteristic analysis: an overview, _Nurse Researcher_ 4(2): 75–88

Bedi A (1993) A tool to fill the gap: developing a wound risk assessment chart for children. _Prof Nurse_ 9(2): 112–20

Cockett A (1998) Paediatric pressure sore risk assessment. _J Tissue Viability_ 8(1): 30

Curley MAQ, Quigley SM, Lin M (2003) Pressure ulcers in pediatric intensive care: incidence and associated factors. _Pediatr Crit Care Med_ 4(3): 284–90

Davis P (1998) The pressure is on: preventing pressure sores. _J Orthopaedic Nurs_ 2(3): 170–6

Dealey C (1991) The size of the pressure-sore problem in a teaching hospital. _J Adv Nurs_ 16(6): 663–70

Deeks J (1996) Pressure sore prevention: using and evaluating risk assessment tools. _Br J Nurs_ 5(5): 313–20

Edwards M (1996a) Pressure sore risk calculators: some methodological issues. _J Clin Nurs_ 5(5): 307–12

Edwards M (1996b) Pressure sore risk: validating an assessment tool. _Br J Community Health Nurs_ 1(5): 282–8

Flanagan M (1995) Who is at risk of a pressure sore? A practical review of risk assessment systems. _Prof Nurse_ 10(5): 305–8

Garvin G (1997) Wound and skin care for the PICU. _Crit Care Nurs Q_ 20(1): 62–71

Gould D (2001) Pressure ulcer risk assessment. _Primary Health Care_ 11(5): 43–9

Groeneveld A, Anderson M, Allen S, Bressmer S, Golberg S, Golberg M *et al* (2004) The prevalence of pressure ulcers in a tertiary care pediatric and adult hospital. *J WOCN* **31**(3): 108–22

Haalboom JRE, den Boer J, Buskens E (1999) Risk assessment tools in the prevention of pressure ulcers. *Ostomy/Wound Management* **45**(2): 20–34

Halfens RJG (2000) Risk assessment scales for pressure ulcers: a theoretical, methodological, and clinical perspective. *Ostomy/Wound Management* **46**(8): 36–44

Huffines B, Logsdon MC (1997) The neonatal skin risk assessment scale for predicting skin breakdown in neonates. *Issues Comprehensive Pediatr Nurs* **20**(2): 103–14

Loman DG (2000) Assessment of skin breakdown risk in children. *J Child Family Nurs* **3**(3): 234–8

MacDonald K (1995) The reliability of pressure sore risk-assessment tools. *Prof Nurse* **11**(3): 169–71

Maylor M, Roberts A (1999) A comparison of three risk assessment scales. *Prof Nurse* **14**(9): 629–32

Olding L, Patterson J (1998) Growing concern. *Nurs Times* **94**(38): 74–9

Pickersgill J (1997) Taking the pressure off. *Paediatr Nurs* **9**(8): 25–7

Samaniego IA (2003) A sore spot in pediatrics: risk factors for pressure ulcers. *Pediatr Nurs* **29**(4): 278–82

Watkinson C (1996) Inter-rater reliability of risk-assessment scales. *Prof Nurse* **11**(11): 751–6

Waterlow J (1998) Pressure sores in children: risk assessment. *Paediatr Nurs* **10**(4): 22–3

Waterlow J (1997) Pressure sore risk assessment in children. *Paediatr Nurs* **9**(6): 21–4

Waterlow J (1995) Reliability of the Waterlow score. *J Wound Care* **4**(10): 474

Willock J, Harris C, Harrison J, Poole C (2005) Identifying the characteristics of children with pressure ulcers. *Nurs Times* **101**(11): 40–3

Paediatric pressure risk assessment tools

Bedi, 1993		
	Description	**Score**
Weight	Average according to age Below birth weight Below weight according to age Overweight	0 2 3 3
Continence	Continent Catheterised Incontinent for children >4 years Nappies Nappy rash Enuretic	0 1 2 2 3 3
Skin types	Dark Fair Sensitive Broken/spot	0 1 2 3
Mobility	Fully Restless/fidgety Sedated/non-walker/restricted Paralysed	0 1 2 4
Appetite	Average/good Poor NG tube Fluids only Malabsorption Failure to thrive Nil by mouth/dehydrated	0 1 2 2 3 3 3
Age	Neonate Infant Toddler Pre-school (2–5 years) 12 years plus	3 1 1 1 1
General assessment	Severe cyanosis and clubbing Moderate cyanosis Mild cyanosis Asymptomatic	5 3 1 0

Bedi, 1993 *cont*		
	Description	**Score**
Special risks	Tissue malnutrition, eg. terminal cachexia	8
	Circulatory/vascular disease	5
	Diabetes	4
	Hypoxaemia	5
	Inotrope support	3
	Known infection, eg. MRSA, Pseudomonas	2
Neurological deficit	Unconsciousness	5
	Developmentally delayed	2
	Achieved normal milestone	0
Major surgery/ trauma	On table >2 hours	5
	On table >5 hours	7
Medication	Antibiotic-induced diarrhoea/thrush/rashes	3

NG = nasogastric; MRSA = methicillin-resistant *Staphylococcus aureus*

Score classification		
10+ at risk	15+ high risk	20+ very high risk

Cockett, 1998		
	Description	**Score**
Weight	Normal weight	0
	Underweight	2
	Overweight	2
Mobility	Able to move self	1
	Restricted mobility	2
	Immobile	3
Skin condition	Intact	0
	Rashes	2
	Oedema	2
	Broken areas	3
	Extravasation injury	3
Diet	NG/oral feeding	1
	IV fluids only	2
	Restricted fluids	2
	TPN	2
	NBM	2

Cockett, 1998 *cont*		
	Description	**Score**
Sedation	No sedation	0
	Oral sedation	I
	IV sedation	2
	IV paralysis	3
Haemodynamic status	Low inotrope	I
	Medium inotrope	3
	High inotrope	5
	Not applicable	0
Respiratory status	Self-ventilating	0
	CPAP/flow driver	I
	Mechanical ventilation	2
Incontinence	Non/catheterised	0
	Nappies	I
	Incontinent	2
Glasgow coma scale	Score 10–15	0
	Score 5–9	I
	Score less than 5	2
Special considerations	Cooled temperature < 35°C	3
	Surgery > 4 hours	3
	Orthopaedic cast	3
	Splinted limbs (including IV)	3

CPAP = continuous positive airway pressure; IV = intravenous; NBM = nil by mouth; TPN = total parenteral nutrition; Inotrope = a drug which increases the force of cardiac compression, eg. adrenaline, isoprenaline

Garvin, 1997	
	Description
A. Mobility (ability to control and change position)	1. No limitations: Age appropriate activity: makes major and frequent changes in position without assistance
	2. Lightly limited: Makes frequent minor changes in position without assistance, spends majority of day in bed or chair
	3. Very limited: Makes occasional slight changes in body or extremity position but unable to make frequent significant changes independently. Ability to walk severely limited or non-existent. Cannot bear own weight or must be assisted into chair or wheelchair
	4. Completely immobile: Does not make any changes in body position without assistance. Confined to bed

Garvin, 1997 *cont*		
	Description	
B. Sensory perception (the ability to respond meaningfully to pressure-related discomfort)	1.	No impairment: Has no sensory deficit which would limit ability to feel or demonstrate pain or discomfort
	2.	Slightly impaired: Has some sensory impairment which limits the ability to feel pain or discomfort in 1 or 2 extremities
	3.	Very limited: Has sensory impairment which limits the ability to feel pain or discomfort over the body
	4.	Completely immobile: Does not make any changes in body position without assistance. Confined to bed
	5.	Completely limited: Unresponsive to painful stimuli due to diminished level of consciousness or sedation, limited ability to feel pain or discomfort over most of the body
C. Nutrition (nutrition to meet growth needs) oral, tube feeds, or hyperalimen-tation	1.	Excellent: Nutrition intake meets 100% of growth needs
	2.	Adequate: Nutrition that meets 75% of growth needs
	3.	Probably inadequate: Receives less than optimum amount of nutrition for an extended period of time, ie. 3 days in a malnourished patient and possibly 7 days in a previously healthy child
D. Moisture (degree to which skin is exposed to moisture)	1.	Rarely moist: Skin is usually dry
	2.	Occasionally moist: Skin is occasionally moist, routine diaper changes every 2–4 hours.
	3.	Moist: Skin is often but not always moist
	4.	Constantly moist: Skin is kept moist almost constantly by perspiration, urine, medicine, etc. Dampness is detected every time the patient is moved or turned

Patient risk score/intervention category:

4–5	None
6–7	Level I
8–12	Level II
8–14	Patients in rehabilitation unit
13–16	Level III

Intervention categories:

I. Level one: Pressure reduction products, ie. Spenco pad, sheepskin pad, etc
II. Level two: Mattress overlay of 4" foam, or Hill Rom™ Critical care bed
III. Level three: The preferred choice is the RIK™ fluid mattress

The Braden Q pressure ulcer risk assessment tool for children (Loman, 2000)		
Mobility	1. 2. 3. 4.	Completely immobile Very limited Slightly limited No limitations
Activity	1. 2. 3. 4.	Bedfast Chairfast Walks occasionally Patient too young to ambulate, or walks frequently
Sensory perception	1. 2. 3. 4.	Completely limited Very limited Slightly limited No impairment
Moisture	1. 2. 3. 4.	Constantly moist Very moist Occasionally moist Rarely moist
Friction–shear	1. 2. 3. 4.	Significant problem Problem Potential problem No apparent problem
Nutrition	1. 2. 3. 4.	Very poor Inadequate Adequate Excellent
Tissue perfusion and oxygenation	1. 2. 3. 4.	Extremely compromised: Hypotensive (MAP <50 mmHg; <40 in newborn) or the patient does not physiologically tolerate position changes Compromised: Normotensive; oxygen saturation may be <95%, or haemoglobin may be <10 g/l; capillary refill may be >2 seconds; serum pH is <7.40 Adequate: Normotensive; oxygen saturation may be <95%, or haemoglobin may be <10 g/l; capillary refill may be >2 seconds; serum pH is normal Excellent: Normotensive; oxygen saturation may be <95%; normal Hb; capillary refill <2 seconds

Total:

Average scores: 25 points = low risk
21 points = medium risk
16 points = high risk

Pickersgill, 1997

Derbyshire Children's Hospital Paediatric Risk Assessment Score

Build and weight for height		Mobility	
Average	0	Full. Normal for age	0
Above average	1	Restless. Fidgety	1
Obese	2	Moves with limited assistance	2
Below average	3	Dependent on others	3
Appetite		Elimination	
Normal for child	0	Completely continent or	0
Insufficient to maintain weight	2	catheterised	
Poor, eats and drinks little	2	Occasionally incontinent	1
Very poor, unable or refuses	3	Frequently incontinent	2
		Fully incontinent, no control	3
Skin condition		Drugs	
Healthy	0	Cytotoxic drug therapy	3
Clammy (eg. pyrexial)	1	High dose steroids	3
Dry skin, dehydrated, lack of turgor	2	High dose non-steriodal	3
Oedematous	2	anti-inflammatories	
Discoloured	2		
Broken skin	3		

Total risk score:

0–5	Low risk
6–10	Medium risk
11 and above	High risk

The Pattoid pressure scoring system (Olding and Patterson, 1998)

Cardiovascular	1.	Stable without inotrope
	2.	Stable with inotrope support
	3.	Inotrope support and unstable
Thermo-regulation	1.	Normothermic
	3.	Hyperthermic/hypothermic
Respiratory	1.	Self-ventilating in air
	2.	Face mask/head box oxygen
	3.	Intubated
Mobility	1.	Normal mobility
	2.	Restricted mobility
	3.	Paralysed and sedated

The Pattoid pressure scoring system (Olding and Patterson, 1998) *cont*		
Nutrition	1.	Unrestricted diet and fluids
	2.	Fluid restriction as enteral/total parenteral nutrition only
	3.	Fluid restriction
Continence	1.	Fully continent
	2.	Incontinent of faeces only (catheterised)
	3.	Incontinent of urine and faeces (wearing nappies)
Skin condition	1.	Intact
	2.	Oedematous/clinically overloaded/discoloration/ marking easily
	3.	Broken/excoriated/surgical wounds/burns
Weight status	1.	Average
	2.	Overweight
	3.	Underweight

Pressure score:

8–14	Low risk
15–20	Medium risk
20+	High risk

Paediatric pressure sore/skin damage risk assessment form (Waterlow, 1998)
Name ....   Age ....   Sex ....

Instructions

1. Complete on admission
2. Reassess if there are any changes to condition or treatment
3. Answer all questions either ✓ or ✗
4. Consider options available and implement as necessary
5. Record any options used
6. Sign the form

Paediatric pressure sore/skin damage risk assessment form (Waterlow, 1998) *cont*

On admission: ✓ Yes ✗ No

1. Does the child have severe physical difficulties, eg. cerebral palsy?   A D G
2. Head injury   A C D
3. Appears malnourished   A I
4. Appears to be severely ill? eg. meningococcal septicaemia   A/B J
5. Is there any skin damage/bruising present?

Define injuries on 'body map' diagram and consider reporting findings.

Treatment:

1. Intensive care?   A/B C D
2. Ventilated/immobile?   A B F G
3. Major surgery – over 5 hours? eg. transplant surgery   A/B H
4. Plaster cast?   E G
5. Splint?   E G
6. Infusion/drain/nasogastric tubing etc?   G
7. Intensive treatment for malignancy, eg. bone marrow transplant?   A I

Record all injuries/areas of skin damage

A – Overlay
B – Alternating pressure overlay
C – Gel pad with shaped cut-out for ear or occiput
D – Regular turning
E – Skin protection, eg. felt padding
F – Barrier cream
G – Skin protection, eg. semi-occlusive dressing
H – Pressure-reducing table top
I – Food supplements
J – Silk sheets

ASSESSOR: ....

DATE OF ASSESSMENT: ....

CHAPTER 6

PREVENTION OF PRESSURE ULCERS IN CHILDREN

Krzysztof S Gebhardt

In the last ten years acceptance has grown that sick children develop pressure ulcers. This has prompted healthcare organisations to develop policies and guidelines which include children and manufacturers of anti-pressure ulcer devices to produce paediatric equipment. In both areas, lack of reliable evidence has been a problem.

The evidence base for pressure ulcer prevention in adults is narrow. For children it is fair to say that it is virtually non-existent. The development and use of pressure-relieving devices highlights some of the dilemmas our limited knowledge raises. Alternating pressure devices, provided they are large-celled (depth 10 cm+) and mechanically reliable, have been shown to be effective in most adult groups. Small-celled have proved generally ineffective. In children, the findings relating to depth may be irrelevant because of the differences in body size. In adults, with the exception of complex flotation devices, constant low pressure devices have not proved to be effective outside of orthopaedics. That does not mean, again due to different weight and morphology, that they will be ineffective in children.

Anecdotal evidence suggests that both approaches may be effective in preventing pressure ulcers in paediatric critical care. Indeed, it would appear that with the introduction of alternating and non-alternating pressure air mattresses in this setting, numbers of ulcers on support surfaces may decline. The real challenge has become reduction of iatrogenic damage, caused by oxygen masks, nasal cannulae, catheters, etc. This may prove a more difficult challenge in the long run.

When we first suggested including paediatric wards in the pressure ulcer (PU) monitoring being carried out in my large teaching trust, there was a lot of opposition. The basis of this opposition was that it would be a waste of time, since children 'do not develop pressure ulcers'. Nevertheless, the manager for paediatrics and I persisted and we discovered that although incidence varied, the numbers were not insignificant. Not surprisingly, the majority of ulcers occurred in the paediatric intensive care unit (PICU), and the overall number of children affected grew when the unit expanded between 1996–1997 (*Figure 6.1*).

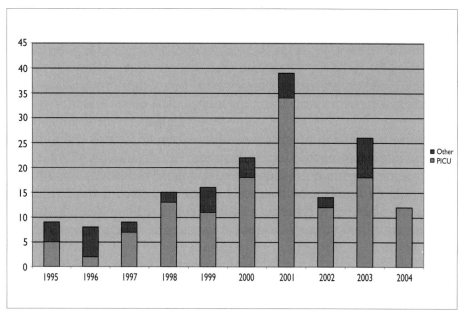

Figure 6.1: The number of pressure ulcers per annum in the paediatric intensive care unit and other paediatric wards

These results indicated that failure to provide pressure area care for children was unacceptable. However, at that time (1995–1997), developing a policy and finding suitable pressure-relieving equipment was difficult. There were no readily available guidelines, there was little or no discussion of the issue, and even if a straightforward translation of policy for adults was attempted, the availability of suitable tools and resources was limited in the extreme. A member of the paediatric nursing team developed a risk assessment tool (Cockett, 1998) and, working with industry, we helped in the development of an alternating pressure air mattress. Since that time, interest in the subject and, with it, the range of tools and equipment has grown. However, as is generally the case with pressure ulcer prevention, serious research interest appears to have been limited. As a result, there seems little to guide the practitioner on how to set about preventing pressure ulcers in children, beyond opinion and accepted practice.

Pressure ulcer prevention

Assessment

The first step in any preventive endeavour is to identify individuals who are at sufficiently high risk to warrant intervention. It seems reasonable to expect PU assessment to take place within two hours of the patient being admitted to an acute care setting. Bearing in mind that even if assessment is acted upon immediately, it is likely to be up to two hours before appropriate equipment can be put in place. That means that even in the best run hospital, the patient may be without mechanical pressure relief for four hours from admission, and may have spent quite some time previously without any pressure area care at all. Time is, therefore, crucial.

This may well be even more important in children than in adults. Pressure ulcers are, in essence, acute ischaemic injuries. As such, they are likely to occur more rapidly when the metabolic rate of the tissues affected, is high. Therefore, it is not unreasonable to assume that with their comparatively high metabolic rate, very young and susceptible children would be particularly vulnerable to rapid onset of pressure damage. In other words, if pressure ulcers do occur in children, they are likely to develop more quickly. It seems reasonable to argue that in an area where the vast majority of patients are susceptible (such as paediatric critical care), preventive protocols should be instigated routinely (including provision of pressure-relieving devices) without necessarily waiting to carry out assessment so that there is no delay in provision. Formal pressure ulcer risk assessment can be carried out later when the patient has been stabilised and pressure-relieving devices, for example, can be removed if unnecessary. In effect, an opt-out rather than an opt-in system may be best.

Repositioning

It could be assumed that repositioning 'at-risk' children might be easier than with adults as they tend to be smaller and lighter. However, this is an oversimplification. Since children have a faster metabolic rate, they are likely to need more frequent turning for the same pressure-relieving effect. When relying on repositioning to provide pressure area protection, it is usually forgetting to turn patients on time, or the inability to do so due to other priorities which leads to development of PUs, rather than the practical difficulties of repositioning *per se*. Needing more frequent repositioning, children would be particularly vulnerable to such failures of repositioning schedules.

Furthermore, some children are not so light! With the growing tide of childhood obesity, some paediatric patients may well weigh as much as, or even more than, average adults. We have nursed at least one 12-year-old on a mattress replacement system as he weighed in excess of 100 kg. More importantly, most susceptible children are in critical care areas. It is impossible to reposition many of these as they are simply too unstable to move. For these and other reasons, mechanical pressure-relieving devices are just as essential for pressure area care in children as in adults.

Pressure-relieving equipment

There has been a growing belief since the 1960s that pressure-relieving/reducing supports are a valuable component of pressure ulcer prevention (Bliss *et al*, 1966). Indeed, it is generally accepted nowadays that they are effective (National Institute for Health and Clinical Excellence [NICE], 2001), and that all patients at risk should be provided with them (Modernisation Agency, 2003).

Pressure-relieving devices fall into two categories. Constant low pressure (CLP) devices aim to distribute pressure as evenly as possible to prevent high pressure points. There is a wide range of these devices from simple sheepskins and foam mattresses with various surface configurations, to complex air-fluidised bead and low airloss bed systems. Pressure-redistributing devices are divided into two further categories. Turning beds and mattresses reposition the patient bodily by tilting or levering him/her from one position to another. Alternating pressure (AP) mattresses cyclically inflate and deflate sets of air cells thus shifting pressure points from one part of the body to another, allowing sufficient time between shifts for the tissues previously subjected to pressure to recover fully before the next application of pressure. Paediatric versions of most pressure-relieving mattress types are available nowadays. However, the research evidence base for paediatric pressure-relieving mattresses can be used as a good illustration of the dilemmas posed by the limited evidence base available for the prevention of PUs in children generally.

Dilemmas in the use of anti-pressure ulcer devices in paediatrics

There is little disagreement that the evidence base supporting the use of pressure-relieving devices is narrow (Clark *et al*, 2005). Despite numerous calls for more research, for reasons which are beyond the scope of this chapter, studies into the efficacy of anti-pressure ulcer equipment have declined in number over the last 10 years, rather than increased (Gebhardt, 1998). However, some general trends can be deduced from the available literature. While it may be tempting to extrapolate from the adult evidence to paediatrics, I believe this should be done with extreme caution.

Various CLP devices have proven successful in prevention in a number of trials. These include: water mattresses (Andersen, 1982); bead bolster systems (Goldstone *et al*, 1982); cross-cut foam mattresses (Gray *et al*, 1994); cubed foam mattresses (Hofman *et al*, 1994); variable density and cross-cut foam mattresses (Santy, 1994). In the main, these studies have been carried out in orthopaedic patient populations. Studies of simple CLP devices (especially foam) using non-orthopaedic subjects demonstrated limited effectiveness of these devices in adults (Bliss *et al*, 1966; Daeschel and Conine, 1985; Stapleton, 1986; Stoneberg *et al*, 1986; Conine *et al*, 1990; Lazzara and Buschmann, 1991; Rimmer, 1992; Gebhardt, 1994).

Although the reaction between body and support may be similar in nature, whether the body in question is that of a child or an adult, it is very different in magnitude. Firstly, the smaller the child the greater the surface area relative to the weight and, therefore, the interface pressure will be substantially less per kg body weight than in an adult. Clearly, the smaller the child, the greater the effect. Secondly, with different body morphology, the weight distribution will be different in an adult and a child. This too may affect the pressure-relieving efficacy of CLP supports and particularly pseudo-flotation devices such as static air mattresses. Some anecdotal evidence suggests that the latter may, in fact, be quite effective especially for very young children. However, as few or no controlled studies of the efficacy of such devices have been carried out with children as subjects, the question of their efficacy or otherwise remains an open one.

Alternating pressure (AP) devices (specifically alternating pressure air mattresses [APAMs]) have been the subject of probably more research than any other type of pressure-relieving device. In summary, (and bearing in mind provisos about the quality of the studies concerned [Cullum *et al*, 1995]), the evidence suggests that APAMs are effective provided they are reliable mechanically and of minimum 10 cm depth (Bliss *et al*, 1966; Andersen *et al*, 1982; Gebhardt *et al*, 1994; Bliss, 1995). There is reasonably consistent evidence that mattresses prone to regular mechanical failures are not effective and neither are small-celled devices — those with cells less than 10 cm in diameter, bubble pads, etc (Exton-Smith *et al* 1982; Daeschel and Conine, 1985; Stapleton, 1986; Conine *et al*, 1990; Sideranko *et al* 1992).

However, while adult-sized, large-celled mattresses may be suitable for the older child, this is not the case for younger or under-developed children. The gaps between inflated cells are simply too wide for the smaller body to bridge and it 'falls' into them. The obvious solution is to utilise mattresses whose cell dimensions and separation are scaled-down proportionately to the smaller body. However, this creates a somewhat paradoxical situation of using APAMs on the basis of research carried out in adults but, because of practical limitations, using precisely the equipment that adult research has shown to be ineffective. Our subjective clinical experience with small-celled mattresses (both small-celled 'adult' mattresses and scaled-down 'paediatric' versions) has been good for pressure ulcer prevention, but clinical opinion or even uncontrolled data is not a good substitute for real controlled trial evidence.

Furthermore, the pressures necessary to keep even small bodies from 'bottoming through' the thinner 'paediatric' APAMs are, of necessity, high. This has the effect of making deep imprints in the skin, particularly in oedematous children which can be quite alarming. While this does not appear to cause any problems and, indeed, by in effect 'massaging' the oedematous tissue may even be beneficial due to stimulation of the lymphatic drainage system. However, all these observations are in the realm of theoretical and clinical opinion rather than of clinical evidence. The safety of these products needs to be studied objectively. Questions relating to the impact that placing APAMs in incubators and bassinettes might have on base heating also remain largely unanswered.

Treatment-related pressure ulcers

Looking at the larger picture suggests that what we place at-risk individuals on might be a lesser concern nowadays. Our experience has been that despite increasing numbers of 'at-risk' individuals, the numbers of paediatric patients developing pressure ulcers on their support surfaces is stable or declining slightly. As a percentage, however, the numbers of pressure ulcers caused by medical appliances (such as face masks, catheters, nasal cannulae, etc) seem to be growing. They affect, among other less common sites, the ears, noses, nostrils, foreheads and genitalia (_Figure 6.2_ and _Table 6.1_). Anecdotally, this appears to be a common, if not universal picture, throughout the UK.

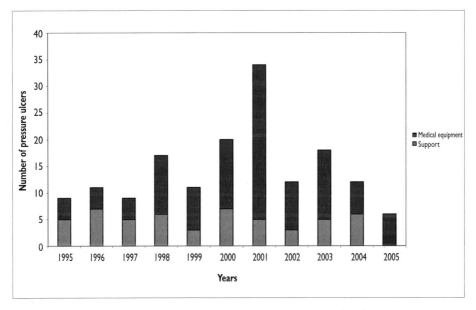

Figure 6.2: Pressure ulcers caused by supports and medical equipment in paediatric critical care

Table 6.1: Anatomical location of ulcers in children and adults in critical care 1995–2005 as a percentage of totals

Location of ulcer	Children, non PICU n=41	PICU n=155	GITU (adults) n=421
Scalp		1.3	
Occiput/head	4.9	5.1	1.4
Cheek		1.3	0.2
Chin		1.3	0.7
Face		1.9	0.2
Mouth		1.3	1.9
Tongue			0.2
Nose		16.1	1.2
Ear	4.8	27.1	2.9
Neck		3.4	1.0
Back	2.4	1.9	1.2
Chest		1.3	
Abdomen			0.2
Arm	4.9	1.9	0.7
Elbow	7.3	0.7	4.3
Wrist	4.9	0.7	0.7
Sacrum/buttocks	48.3	12.9	59.4
Genitals		3.9	1.4
Leg	2.4	0.7	0.2
Thigh		1.9	1.2
Knee	2.4	1.3	1.0
Foot		3.9	1.4
Heel	17.0	7.7	17.8
Toe		1.9	0.5

PICU = paediatric intensive care unit; GITU = general intensive care unit

Analysis of *Table 6.1* shows some interesting trends. Patients in critical care, regardless of age, sustain a wide range of pressure injuries not usually found elsewhere. However, there the similarity ends, as quantitatively the anatomical distribution of ulcers in adult intensive care units (ICUs) seems to have a lot more in common with the distribution in non-critical paediatric patients than with paediatric intensive care units (PICUs). In both cases, most of the damage appears to be related to pressure from support surfaces, with the two most common sites for this type of injury, the sacrum/buttocks and heels, accounting for approximately 65% (non-critical care paediatrics), and nearly 77% in GITU.

While sacral/buttock and heel ulcers are not unimportant in PICU, they only account for just over 20% of the total. On the other hand, ear and nose ulcers (many of them affecting the nostrils) are the most common ulcers accounting for nearly half. Ear and nose ulcers do occur in the other two groups, but are comparatively rare making up less than 5% in both groups. Some of these injuries are relatively unique to children because their heads are proportionately larger to their body size — ear ulcers are twice as common in non-PICU children as they are in GITU adults — nevertheless, it seems probable that most of these injuries are caused by the application of oxygen masks and nasal cannulae in PICU.

As one would expect, there are also some similarities between pressure ulcer distribution in non-critical and critical paediatric care. For example, ulcers to the back and sides of the head, most likely related to the comparatively large head of the infant, are 3.5 times as likely in children as they are in GITU adults. While this area of risk should be considered by healthcare professionals caring for children, pressure ulcers in these areas only account for around 5% of the total in both cases.

Conclusions

Pressure ulcer prevention in children has risen rapidly in importance and profile over the last decade. Industry has responded with the introduction of a wide range of pressure ulcer prevention products. Incidence rates suggest that despite apparently increasing acuity and dependence of paediatric patients, at least some of these products are quite effective. That said, there is little or no reliable research evidence to support their use at present.

However, it is also becoming apparent that in paediatric critical care, which accounts for the majority of pressure ulcers in children, ulcers resulting from contact with the support surface are a relatively small part of the problem. It is, in fact, medical appliances pressing against vulnerable bodies which are causing the most damage. Thus, even though the need for better evidence for the use of pressure-

relieving supports for children might be pressing, the first objectives
of research and development in paediatric pressure area care may well
be the development of better medical appliances. In particular, this
should include new face masks, nasal cannulae and nasogastric tube-
retaining systems, as well as changing accepted practice. These may
prove difficult challenges.

References

Andersen KE, Jensen O, Kvorning SA, Bach E (1982) Decubitus
    prophylaxis: a prospective trial on the efficacy of alternating-pressure
    air-mattresses and water mattresses. *Acta Dermatovenearologica*
    (Stockholm) **63**: 227–30
Bliss MR (1995) Preventing pressure sores in elderly patients – a
    comparison of seven mattress overlays. *Age Ageing* **24**: 297–302
Bliss MR, McLaren R, Exton-Smith AN (1966) Mattresses for preventing
    pressure sores in geriatric patients. *Med Bull Ministry of Health* **25**:
    238–67
Clark M, Hiskett G, Russell L (2005) Evidence-based practice and support
    surfaces: are we throwing the baby out with the bath water? *J Wound
    Care* **14**(10): 455–8
Cockett A (1998) Paediatric pressure sores risk assessment. *J Tissue
    Viability* **8**(1): 30
Conine TA, Daechsel D, Lau MS (1990) The role of alternating air and
    Silicore overlays in preventing decubitus ulcers. *Int J Rehab Res* **13**:
    57–65
Cullum N, Deaks J, Fletcher A, Long A, Mouneimne H, Sheldon T *et al*
    (1995) The prevention and treatment of pressure sores. *Effective Health
    Care* **2**(1)
Daeschel D, Conine TA (1985) Special mattresses: effectiveness in
    preventing decubitus ulcers in chronic neurologic patients. *Arch Phys
    Med Rehabil* **66**: 246–8
Exton-Smith An, Overstall PW, Wedgewood J, Wallace G (1982) Use of
    the 'air-wave' system to prevent pressure sores in hospital. *Lancet* ii:
    1288–90
Gebhardt KS (1994) A randomised trial of alternating pressure (AP) and
    constant low pressure (CLP) supports for the prevention of pressure
    sores. *J Tissue Viability* **4**(3): 93

Gebhardt KS (1998) Editorial. *J Tissue Viability* 8(4): 2

Goldstone L, Norris M, O'Reilly M, White J (1982) A clinical trial of a bead bed system for the prevention of pressure sores in elderly orthopaedic patients. *J Adv Nurs* 7: 545–8

Gray DG, Campbell M (1994) A randomised clinical trial of two types of foam mattresses. *J Tissue Viability* 4: 128–32

Hofman A, Geelkerken RH, Hamming JJ (1994) Pressure sores and pressure decreasing mattresses: controlled clinical trial. *Lancet* 343: 568–71

Lazzara DJ, Buschmann MBT (1991) Prevention of pressure ulcers in elderly nursing home residents: are special support surfaces the answer? *Decubitus* 4: 42–6

Modernisation Agency (2003) *Essence of Care. Patient-focused benchmarks for clinical governance.* Modernisation Agency, London

National Institute for Health and Clinical Excellence (2001) *Inherited clinical guideline B. Pressure ulcer risk assessment and prevention.* NICE, London

Rimmer C (1992) Establishing the cost of comfort: effectiveness of mattresses in pressure sore prevention. *Prof Nurse* Sept: 810–15

Santy JE, Butler MK, Whyman JD (1994) A comparison study of 6 types of hospital mattress to determine which most effectively reduces the incidence of pressure sores in elderly patients with hip fractures in a district general hospital. Unpublished report to Northern and Yorkshire Regional Health Authority

Sidernako S, Quinn A, Burns K, Froman RD (1992) Effects of position and mattress overlay on sacral and heel pressures in a clinical population. *Res Nurs Health* 15: 245–51

Stapleton M (1986) Preventing pressure sores – an evaluation of three products. *Geriatr Nurs* 6: 23–5

Stoneberg C, Pitcock N, Myton C (1986) Pressure sores in the homebound: one solution. *Am J Nurs* 86: 426–8

CHAPTER 7

INFANT NAPKIN DERMATITIS AND DIFFERENTIAL DIAGNOSES

Richard White and Jacqueline Denyer

Skin problems are common in infants, with irritant dermatitis of the napkin area being the most common, affecting from a quarter to one third of the at-risk age group (Odio, 2000; Shin, 2005). To understand how and why this disorder arises, and how to manage it, it is first important to gain an understanding of the skin of the neonate. Thereafter, skin care, washing, napkin changing and selection all become central to management or avoidance (Atherton, 2004).

This chapter includes a review of our current knowledge of irritant napkin (diaper) dermatitis (IND), including causative mechanisms, skin maceration, barrier treatments and skin emollients, cleansing and use of soaps, choosing nappies, and, in established IND, topical medications.

The skin of the neonate will vary in structure and functional capacity depending on the gestational age at birth, and the body site (Yosipovitch *et al*, 2006). Those variables relating to skin barrier function, namely stratum corneum hydration, pH and transepidermal water loss (TEWL), show significant differences from adult skin. Now that we have the capability of sustaining life from about 24 weeks gestational age, care must be taken to protect those organs that are not fully functional at the time of birth — this includes the skin (*Chapters 1* and *2*). Neonatal skin, particularly in the crural/inguinal area, is highly hydrated, has a high pH (ie. over 6; Gfatter *et al*, 1997), and is susceptible to irritants (Shin, 2005). In view of the relatively high skin surface pH, the use of alkaline soaps and detergents is not recommended as it will compromise the formation of the protective 'acid mantle' of the skin (Gfatter *et al*, 1997; Rippke *et al*, 2002; Yosipovitch, 2006).

Irritant napkin (diaper) dermatitis: Presentation and aetiology

Although IND is most often seen in the 9–12-month-age group (Jordan _et al_, 1986), it can manifest much earlier with an onset around 3–4 weeks. There is no difference in prevalence reported between gender or race (USA data: Ward _et al_, 2000). The most common form is an irritant dermatitis, ie. a skin reaction resulting from non-immunologic damage by chemicals in contact with the skin. The common predisposing factors are:

- friction
- moisture
- urine
- faeces
- microorganisms
- diet.

A combination of more than one of these factors usually exists (Scheinfeld, 2005).

Aetiology

Predisposing factors

- ❖ _Maceration of the crural/inguinal area:_ the skin can become macerated from excess hydration either by TEWL or by exposure to urine.
- ❖ _Occlusion of the crural area:_ prolonged occlusion of the skin can itself produce erythema due to increased sweating and TEWL.
- ❖ _Water:_ hydration and friction may be responsible for many cases of napkin dermatitis making the skin more susceptible to irritants. It has been suggested that prolonged contact with water alone can provoke dermatitis. Maceration of the stratum corneum by water may be an important predisposing factor, which increases transepidermal permeability, friction and infections.

* *Urine:* the role of urine in precipitating the skin lesions may be due to increased pH or higher contents of ammonia. This may explain the findings that breast-fed infants are less liable to IND than those fed on cows' milk (Berg *et al*, 1986; Benjamin, 1987). In addition, urine appears to increase transepidermal permeability more effectively than water alone. This might be due to the proteolytic action of urea.

* *Faeces:* human faeces have an irritant effect on skin. Infants' faeces contain substantial amounts of pancreatic protease and lipase. Similar enzymes appear to be produced within the gut by a variety of bacteria, causing irritation and leading to higher pH of faeces. One of the factors that have been shown to affect faecal pH is the infant's diet (Buckingham and Berg, 1986). Higher pH faeces being found in cows' milk and formula-fed infants.

* *Friction:* friction between the skin and the fabric of the nappy plays at least some part in the aetiology.

* *Microorganisms:* the most frequent pathogen associated with nappy rash is *Candida albicans*. This organism is usually sensitive to imidazole antifungal agents such as clotrimazole 1%. Super-infection with candida is strongly associated with the increased wetness caused by non-breathable nappies (Akin *et al*, 2001). The use of broad-spectrum oral antibiotics increases the recovery of *Candida albicans* from the rectum and skin; this will aggravate primary irritant napkin dermatitis (Rebora and Leyden, 1981).

* *Chemical irritants:* soaps, detergents and antiseptics used to clean washable napkins have often been incriminated in the initiation and aggravation of primary irritant napkin dermatitis.

* *Obesity:* obese infants are more susceptible to IND.

Clinical features

Nappy rash is a generic term for a range of conditions affecting the crural/inguinal area. The classification of skin reactions includes IND, candida infection, infantile seborrhoeic eczema, atopic eczema, noduloulcerative nappy dermatitis, intertrigo and others (Rasmussen, 1987).

Skin lesions and the various presentations of nappy rash

IND presents as a confluent erythema of the area in contact with the nappy, ie. the crural area of buttocks, genitalia, lower abdomen, pubic area and upper thighs. In some infants, the eruption is more or less confined to the margins of the napkin area. Before making a diagnosis of nappy rash, we should consider its different guises, namely:

❖ *Acute lesions:* the erythema may have a glazed appearance, where later there may be exfoliation of the affected areas of the skin.
❖ *Chronic cases:* these show finer scaling.
❖ *Erythematous type:* this appears as intensely red confluent erythema of the entire perineal area, including the depths of the flexural folds. Skin lesions present with erythema and slightly elevated margins. Within the marginal area, small pustules may involve the periphery of the erythema — so-called 'satellite' lesions. This clinical type is associated with more intense proliferation of *Candida albicans* and is invariably associated with faecal carriage of this organism.
❖ *Psoriasiform type:* the erythematous areas are similarly well marginated but have a psoriasiform aspect with prominent scaling. The onset of this eruption is commonly termed 'napkin psoriasis' that may be quite sudden and its extension is rapid.
❖ *Herpetiform type:* this takes the form of an eruption of vesicles and pustules followed by shallow erosions, and closely resembles herpes simplex clinically, but showing no evidence of this infection pathologically (Graham-Brown *et al*, 1986).
❖ *Granulomatous type:* this rare type manifests with dome-shaped, reddish-brown or purple nodules. The lesions are usually known as infantile gluteal granuloma.
❖ *Extensive type:* the lesion extends peripherally to include the lower abdomen and back which may reach the axillary folds. Some believe that it is a manifestation of infantile seborrhoeic dermatitis.
❖ *Hypopigmented type:* post-inflammatory hypopigmentation may be a striking feature in racially-pigmented infants.
❖ *Erosive type:* this appears in primary irritant napkin dermatitis. Small vesicles and erosions may develop into rather characteristic shallow round ulcers with raised crater-like edge. Involvement of the genitalia may lead to dysuria. If the glans penis is severely affected, male infants may experience acute retention of urine.

Treatments

Successful treatment of napkin dermatitis depends mainly on detection of the predisposing factors and implementing corrective measures. The application of topical medications alone, without correction of the predisposing factors, is often rewarded with a therapeutic failure. As a general rule, frequent changing of absorbent, breathable nappies, combined with careful skin hygiene, are the most essential measures.

Considerations about nappies

When disposable nappies are not available, the washable type can be used. Care should be taken concerning the washable nappies in order to give the best results. These include the type of cloth: this should be made of soft, absorbent cotton (eg. Terry towelling). Many modern, washable nappies are made from polyester fleece — this allows rapid passage of urine through to a highly absorptive inner layer, leaving the surface next to the skin almost dry.

The absorbency of the napkin is another important factor (Stein, 1982). Washable cloth napkins have the advantage of allowing two or more layers to be worn at once to increase the volume of urine that can be effectively absorbed. As the baby becomes older, though the frequency of urination falls, the volume voided on each occasion rises.

Wash with mild soap, not biological powder, and rinse thoroughly to remove any remnants of detergents. The enzymes in biological powders are known to be allergenic (Flindt, 1995; 1996). Avoid fabric conditioners and bleach.

Disposable nappies are available in different types and with different absorbent efficiency. A suitable size according to the age of the infant should be used in order not to compress the skin of the thighs and abdomen.

Care of nappies

The use of antiseptic solutions for the storage of napkins prior to washing is more or less universal (eg. Milton®). These may be safe as long as used according to manufacturers' instructions (http://www.

milton-tm.com/docs/milton_hygiene_guide.pdf) and rinsing procedures are adequate. Toxicity from antiseptics used in the laundry washing of napkins is well documented (Shin, 2005).

The quaternary ammonium compounds are now regarded as the best choice, of which benzalkonium chloride is perhaps the most widely employed. Antiseptics should never be used during the rinsing process.

Changing nappies

The frequency of nappy changes is almost certainly more important than either the type used, or the wearing of occlusive over-pants. Routine changing, or at least checking the nappy for wetting or soiling at regular periods, is essential.

Preventive measures

Effective treatment is directed mainly at preventing irritation and towards the predisposing factors.

Avoid using wipes for cleaning the skin, especially those soaked with alcohol, antiseptics or perfume. Gentle cleaning of the diaper area is important. Use mild, non-irritating, non-perfumed soap. Excessively meticulous cleaning will do more harm. Rubbing the area should be avoided. Cleaning with a mild soap and a soft sponge is all that is needed.

At each napkin change, an emollient such as white soft paraffin, or a 50/50 mixture of white soft paraffin and liquid paraffin, or zinc and castor oil cream BP should be applied if the napkin has not been wetted or soiled.

If the napkin has been wetted or soiled, the area should be cleansed with water and a water-miscible emollient application, such as emulsifying ointment BP, and dried before applying a water-repellent emollient.

The use of talc and over-the-counter preparations containing potential irritants should be discouraged.

Cleaning infant skin

The ideal cleanser for neonates and infants should:

- be delicate, 'skin-friendly' with pH-balanced surfactants
- not contain perfumes (frequent sensitisers)
- not contain alcohol (causes stinging)
- not contain substances known to cross-react with other allergens.

It is important that the crural area is left exposed and free for some time daily, without nappies, for aeration.

Rubber or plastic panties worn over the nappy should be avoided, or used with care, since these may cause more occlusion.

Powders, such as talc and dusting powder, should be avoided if the area is macerated as they may be abrasive and cause irritation. When mixed with moisture, 'caking' occurs forming focal points for trauma and further irritation.

Active treatment

Treatment depends on the type of the lesion of the area. Non-steroidal topical preparations are the first line of treatment. Corticosteroids should be reserved for the most severe, reluctant types of atopic dermatitis, when the non-steroidal preparation fails to clear the lesions. Fluorinated or potent/very potent steroids should be avoided (Harper, 1988; *Chapter 8, Table 8.1, pp. 126–127*). Topical antihistamines should not be used.

Treatments of nappy rash

Wet and macerated nappy area

Excess moisture, dampness and maceration can usually be cleared by more frequent nappy changes and the use of 'super-absorbent' disposable nappies (Sires and Mallory, 1995).

Secondarily-infected lesions

These include species of staphylococcus, streptococcus and enteric anaerobes. Oral antibiotic treatment following culture and sensitivity may be required if topical treatments fail, or the infant is systemically unwell. Consider antifungal treatment in conjunction with antibiotic therapy due to the high risk of candida.

Complicated lesions

Topical antifungal/antimycotic agents, such as clotrimazole 1%, are generally safe and effective in the treatment of candida infections (Lambe, 2001). Some preparations, especially miconazole, may cause local contact allergy reactions provoking more erythema and irritation to the crural areas (Raulin and Frosch, 1988). This reaction may be due to the vehicle causing more irritation to the macerated sensitive skin of the crural area and, in particular, the genitalia.

Antifungal preparations, especially those combined with steroids, should be avoided unless there are compelling reasons for their use. These should be used cautiously and for a short period.

It should be considered that diseased or abraded skin, or occlusive conditions, will considerably enhance the rate of percutaneous absorption of corticosteroids from a topical application (Turpeinen, 1988), especially in the napkin area.

Abuse of topical steroids (using for too long or using too strong a steroid), and occlusion of steroids (plastic pants are occlusive), will increase the risks of hypothalamic-pituitary-adrenal (HPA) axis suppression and skin atrophy in infants. It is also important to exercise extra care when selecting and using topical steroids on particularly vulnerable areas, such as the face and the crural area (Clement and Du Vivier, 1987). Corticosteroids classed as 'mild' or 'moderate' potency (*Chapter 8, Table 8.1, pp. 126–127*) should only be used if the child has eczema which has extended over the nappy area.

Differential diagnoses

Candidiasis

Candidiasis is caused by the opportunistic pathogen *Candida spp*, mainly *albicans*. It has characteristic mucocutaneous clinical features in infants; the presentation varies with site. The typical skin lesions are confluent glistening, sharply marginated and erythematous with peripheral desquamation which may be accompanied by pustulation. Satellite papulopustules are common. Oral candidiasis presents as white, adherent plaques on the mucous membranes. Treatment should be based on accurate diagnosis and involve selected topical antifungals for cutaneous disease (Elewski, 1996).

In neonatal candidiasis, superficial candida infection can be transmitted to the baby during birth. The rash normally appears during the second week of life. While superficial candidiasis is often trivial, in low birth weight neonates (particularly below 750 g), and in the neonatal infection control unit (ICU), invasive infection can be a major cause of morbidity, even life-threatening (Smith *et al*, 2005).

Zinc deficiency

Zinc deficiency (*Acrodermatitis enteropathica*) must be considered in any infant with a napkin dermatitis which fails to respond to appropriate treatment. A history of prematurity should increase suspicion, and a normal plasma zinc level does not rule out the diagnosis.

Infants with napkin eruptions caused by zinc deficiency present with:

- concurrent facial dermatitis extending from the peri-oral area
- an erosive paronychia
- erosions of palmar creases of the hands.

Histiocytosis

Napkin dermatitis is one of the most common skin lesions of Langerhans cell histiocytosis in infants (Sires and Mallory, 1995).

Dermatophyte infections

Tinea cruris (a pruritic superficial fungal infection of the groin and adjacent skin) can be differentiated by the active raised edges, central clearing of lesions, and by detecting the causative organism. Antifungal agents topically, possibly with corticosteroids used cautiously, are known to bring rapid symptom relief (Van Esso *et al*, 1995; Erbagci, 2004).

Herpes simplex virus infection

The eruption is acute, has characteristic painful grouped vesicular lesions on an erythematous base, and is accompanied by constitutional manifestations such as fever.

Neglect

Nappy rash may be associated with general neglect of the infant. Infrequent changes of napkin, together with lack of cleansing, will result in extensive diaper rash. Other signs of neglect, such as failure to thrive and developmental delay in areas of physical ability and social and emotional well-being, may be present.

Child abuse

Deliberate scalding of the buttocks and genitalia can occur in response to aggressive cleansing, for example, holding the child under running hot water. Skin-inflicted injuries must be considered when the history is inconsistent with the child's development, or does not explain the injury (Kairys *et al*, 2002).

There are also a number of relatively unique clinical skin diseases that may develop on the buttocks of infants. These include:

- iatrogenic skin diseases
- skin tumours
- atrophy of the skin due to corticosteroids
- nevi and tumour diseases, such as *nevoxanthoendothelioma* (juvenile xanthogranuloma) and Letterer-Siwe disease (Letterer-Siwe disease is an acute disseminated form of Langerhans cell histiocytosis, occurring most often in children younger than 3 years old. This condition needs to be distinguished from the clinically similar but exceedingly rare disorder of haemophagocytic reticulosis, which often has a familial incidence)
- chronic granulomatous disease (Honda, 1991).

Diarrhoea

Faecal proteolytic enzymes and water are both increased with diarrhoea. These can quickly damage the skin if not washed off.

The possible causes of diarrhoea include:

- infective causes such as viral, bacterial and parasitic, non-enteric infections including otitis media, respiratory and urinary tract infections
- malabsorption resulting from diseases such as coeliac and cystic fibrosis
- food allergy or intolerance
- antibiotic use (Campbell *et al*, 1988)
- immune deficiency. Persistent chronic diarrhoea is a common feature in children who are immune deficient, and particularly those who are positive for human immunodeficiency virus (HIV), or suffering from acquired immune deficiency syndrome (AIDS).

References

Akin F, Spraker M, Aly R *et al* (2001) Effects of breathable, disposable diapers: reduced prevalence of Candida and common diaper dermatitis. *Pediatr Dermatol* 18(4): 282–90

Atherton DJ (2004) A review of the pathophysiolgy, prevention and treatment of irritant diaper dermatitis. *Curr Med Res Opin* 20(5): 645–9

Benjamin L (1987) Clinical correlates with diaper dermatitis. *Pediatrician* 14: 21–6

Berg RW, Buckingham KW, Stewart RL (1986) Etiologic factors in diaper dermatitis: The role of urine. *Pediatr Dermatol* 3: 102–6

Buckingham KW, Berg RW (1986) Etiologic factors in diaper dermatitis: the role of feces. *Pediatr Dermatol* 3: 107–12

Campbell RL, Bartlett AV, Sarbargh FC *et al* (1988) Effect of diaper types on diaper dermatitis associated with diarrhoea and antibiotic use in children and day-care centres. *Pediatr Dermatol* 5: 83–7

Clement M, Du Vivier A (1987) *Topical Steroids for Skin Disorders.* Blackwell Scientific Publications, Oxford

Elewski BE (1996) Cutaneous mycoses in children. *Br J Dermatol* 134(Suppl 46): 7–11

Erbagci Z (2004) Topical therapy for dermatophytoses. *Am J Clin Dermatol* 5(6): 375–84

Flindt ML (1995) Biological washing powders as allergens. *Br Med J* 310(6979): 603

Flindt ML (1996) Biological miracles and misadventures: identification of sensitization and asthma in enzyme detergent workers. *Am J Ind Med* 29(1): 1–2

Gfatter R, Hackl P, Braun F (1997) Effects of soap and detergents on skin surface pH, stratum corneum hydration and fat content in infants. *Dermatology* 195: 258–62

Graham-Brown RA, Lister DM, Burns DA (1986) Herpetiform napkin dermatitis: napkin dermatitis simulating an acute herpes simplex infection. *Br J Dermatol* 114(6): 746–7

Harper J (1988) Topical corticosteroids for skin disorders in infants and children. *Drugs* 36(Suppl 5): 34–7

Honda M (1991) Differential diagnosis of unusual skin diseases in infants. *Arch Dermatol* 127(3): 396–8

Jordan WE, Lawson KD, Berg RW *et al* (1986) Diaper dermatitis: frequency and severity among a general infant population. *Pediatr Dermatol* 3: 198–207

Kairys SW, Alexander RC, Block RW, Everrett UD, Hymel KP, Jenny C, Stirling Jr J (2002) When inflicted skin injuries constitute child abuse. *J Am Acad Pediatr* **110**(3): 644–5

Lambe MB (2001) Topical agents in infants. *Newborn and Infant Nursing Reviews* **1**(1): 25–34

Odio M, Frielander SF, Railan D *et al* (2000) Diaper dermatitis and advances in diaper technology. *Curr Opin Pediatr* **12**(4): 342–6

Rasmussen JE (1987) Classification of diaper dermatitis: an overview. *Pediatrician* **14**(Suppl 1): 6–10

Raulin C, Frosch PJ (1988) Contact allergy to imidazole antimycotics. *Contact Dermatitis* **18**(2): 76–80

Rebora A, Leyden JJ (1981) Napkin (diaper) dermatitis and the gastrointestinal carriage of *Candida albicans*. *Br J Dermatol* **105**(5): 551–55

Rippke F, Schreiner V, Schwanitz HJ (2002) The acid milieu of the horny layer: new findings on the physiology and pathophysiology of skin pH. *Am J Clin Dermatol* **3**(4): 261–72

Scheinfeld N (2005) Diaper dermatitis: a review and brief survey of eruptions of the diaper area. *Am J Clin Dermatol* **6**(5): 273–81

Shin HT (2005) Diaper dermatitis that does not quit. *Dermatologic Therapy* **18**: 124–35

Sires UI, Mallory SB (1995) Diaper dermatitis. How to treat and prevent. *Postgrad Med* **98**(6): 79–84

Smith PB, Steinbach WJ, Benjamin DK (2005) Neonatal candidiasis. *Infect Dis Clin North Am* **19**(3): 603–15

Stein H (1982) Incidence of diaper rash when using cloth and disposable diapers. *J Pediatr* **101**: 720–3

Turpeinen M (1988) Influence of age and severity of dermatitis on the percutaneous absorption of hydrocortisone in children. *Br J Dermatol* **118**(4): 517–22

Van Esso D, Fajo G, Losada I *et al* (1995) Sertaconazole in the treatment of pediatric patients with cutaneous dermatophyte infections. *Clin Ther* **17**(2): 264–9

Ward DB, Fleischer AB, Feldman SR *et al* (2000) Characterization of diaper dermatitis in the United States. *Arch Pediatr Adolesc Med* **154**(9): 943–6

Yosipovitch G, Maayan-Metzger A, Merlob P, Sirota L (2000) Skin barrier properties in different body areas in neonates. *Pediatrics* **106**(1): 105–10

CHAPTER 8

MANAGEMENT OF ATOPIC ECZEMA IN CHILDREN

Rosemary Turnbull

Atopic eczema is a chronic, relapsing inflammatory skin condition associated with epidermal dysfunction (Brown and Reynolds, 2006). It is a distressing, intensely pruritic inflammatory disease affecting both the epidermis and dermis. It generally manifests from around three months of age, although can occur at any age. There is no cure, but 75% of those affected will be clear of the disease by their teens.

The British Association of Dermatologists and the Royal College of Physicians have identified the following diagnostic criterion for atopic eczema (McHenry *et al*, 1995). It must have:

❖ An itchy skin condition (or reported scratching or rubbing in a child).

Plus three or more of the following:

❖ History of itchiness in skin creases, such as fold of the elbows, behind the knees, front of ankles or around the neck (or the cheeks in children under four years).
❖ History of asthma or hayfever (or a history of atopic disease in the first-degree relative in children under four years).
❖ General dry skin in the past year.
❖ Visible, flexural eczema (or eczema affecting the cheeks or forehead and outer limbs in children under four years).
❖ Onset in the first two years of life (not always diagnostic in children under four years).

If there is no itch it is unlikely to be atopic eczema.

Pathophysiology

The aetiology of eczema is multifactorial, with genetic, environmental, immunological and physiological factors, all playing a role in its development. There is also a genetic predisposition to the production of increased levels of IgE antibodies, with a tendency to develop one or more of a group of disorders, such as hayfever, asthma, allergy and urticaria (Harper, 1990).

The epidermis has an inability to hold water and is, therefore, porous, leaking fluid from the cells. This is because individual corneocytes separate, thus reducing epidermal lipids. It is this that makes the skin chronically dry, and the skin barrier less effective (Cork, 1997). This, in turn, allows bacteria to penetrate, which can result in an inflammatory process. This inflammation causes erythema and oedema in the epidermis (spongiosis). The increased blood flow causes leakage of white blood cells into the dermis, heralding the formation of vesicles and blisters in the epidermis which, when scratched, result in wet, weepy eczematous skin.

As said, there is no known cure for this skin condition and the emphasis is on controlling exacerbations and promoting a good quality of life for the child.

Clinical presentation

In infancy, the eczema presents from around three months of age and is predominantly facial with a tendency to being vesicular, wet and weeping. It generally has a non-specific distribution, with any area of the body being affected. The infant will frequently be fractious and wriggles and squirms in an effort to relieve pruritus.

As the child matures, the eczema tends to settle in the limb flexures. The skin is often dry and flaky with extensive excoriations and demonstrates a leathery appearance (lichenification). These excoriations are commonly seen on the ankles, wrists and flexural areas.

In Afro-Caribbean/Asian skin types, children sometimes show a reverse pattern of extensor eczema and generally more lichenification, as well as a more follicular pattern of eczema (Robinson, 2003). There are often areas of alterations in the skin's pigmentation as a result of post-inflammatory pigment changes and, generally, not from topical steroids as many parents fear.

Atopic eczema that persists into adolescence generally remains prominent in the popliteal and antecubital fossae, as well as around the neck. It is frequently characterised by unsightly lichenification, and infraorbital creases may also be visible. Periodically, the eczema can affect the whole body.

Without a doubt, the most common and distressing aspect of atopic eczema at any age is the intense itching and scratching, which is a reflex action to the itch. It is this action that can often distinguish eczema from other skin conditions (Bridgett _et al_, 1996).

Differential diagnosis

❖ If less than three months of age, consider **_seborrhoeic dermatitis_**. This is characterised by cradle cap spreading to the forehead, eyebrows and skin folds. It is unlikely to be pruritic and, although distressing to the parents, causes no discomfort to the infant.

❖ **_Discoid eczema_**: this is characterised by well-defined, coin-shaped lesions that can be dry and scaly, or wet and crusted. It is generally found on the limbs.

❖ **_Allergic/contact eczema_**: this is characterised by an often-limited distribution of erythematous skin with oozing vesicles. The history will often identify the allergen and it will generally improve when the irritant is removed.

❖ **_Psoriasis_**: this is characterised by dry, flaky skin. There are visible plaques rather than the papulovesicular appearance of eczema, and it is rarely pruritic.

❖ **_Scabies_**: this is characterised by intense pruritus. There is often a rash with secondary infection. The soles of the feet and genitalia should be checked carefully.

To manage eczema effectively, it is imperative that time is taken to ensure that parents have a good understanding of the disease process, the rationale for prescribed treatments, and are conscious to avoid known trigger factors. It is time well spent demonstrating the application of all topical therapies to the carer and the child, where applicable. It is also useful to reiterate that there is no cure for eczema, and that the emphasis is on control.

Parents may be extremely anxious and confused about child health facts. It is a good idea to have a structured assessment format which will allow you to gain the optimum amount of information required to assist in the assessment, planning, and implementation of a skin care regime tailored to individual need (see *Appendix* at the end of this chapter, *pp. 131–132*). For younger children, it is useful to ask to see the child health record, as this may offer an insight into the onset of any problem. Accordingly, this booklet should be filled out after the consultation to allow continuity of care and accurate communication between healthcare professionals. It is essential that thorough assessment is carried out if the child is to be treated effectively: eczema is chronic and can have a distressing impact on the child, culminating in an adverse perception of self. Children can be cruel and peers may subject the child to ridicule and exclusion. Depending on the condition, the effect can be equally devastating on the family.

Treatment regimes

The aim of treatment is to hydrate the skin, reduce inflammation, promote comfort, and aim to improve quality of life for the child (Hoare *et al*, 2000).

Bathing

Bathing is required to cleanse and hydrate the skin. Emollient bath oils are an ideal means of introducing moisture into the skin, and should be done on a daily basis. Bathing or showering in water alone can irritate and dry the skin further and so oils should be added. Bath oils are designed to disperse in water, thus coating the skin on entering and leaving the bath.

Bath water should be tepid as, if hot, it will cause vasodilation and increase pruritus. To gain optimum benefit from the emollients, the child should be encouraged to soak in the bath for approximately 15 minutes. Bathing for longer than this can cause the skin to exfoliate and dry out. Bathing is an essential part of eczema management, and the child should be encouraged to have fun using a favourite toy; a selection of washable, bathing toys may go some way to assisting in this.

If there is no access to a bath, an emollient shower gel is advised as well as the use of a soap substitute.

The use of bubble baths must be discouraged, as they contain detergents and fragrances which will strip the natural lipid layer of the skin and cause irritation. If the child gets upset or refuses baths, it may be that they have had a bath without oils and experienced a degree of discomfort.

Care should be taken not to overheat the bathroom as this will also irritate the skin.

The child should not be left unsupervised, as the emollient oils will make the surface of the bath slippery.

Soap

Soaps should be avoided as they contain fragrances and detergents that will remove the natural lipid layer from the skin. The use of soap substitutes in the form of light emollients is encouraged. This will serve to remove dried blood and skin debris. They are best applied to the limbs prior to entering the bath, giving a protective barrier that can sometimes minimise the stinging sensation that some children experience. Emollients can help to reduce skin infection.

Parents need to be informed that soap substitutes do not lather, foam, or have a fragrance.

Emollients

Moisturising of the skin is the main treatment in eczema management. When used frequently and correctly, emollients will have a steroid-sparing effect on eczematous skin. The greasier emollients are the most effective as they are occlusive, forming a good skin barrier (see _Table 8.2, pp. 128–30_). Creams are cosmetically more acceptable but, as they contain many additives, they can cause sensitisation to an already sensitive skin. Choice is key here, as if the parent and/or child do not like their emollient, they will not use it. It is beneficial if more than one is demonstrated to allow the parent/child to choose the one that they prefer — this may take several consultations.

The effects of emollients are short-lived, and if they are to replace the lipid barrier and minimise loss of water through evaporation, they need to be applied frequently throughout the day. They should be applied to the skin quickly and gently in a downward motion in the direction of hair growth, to minimise plugging of the hair follicles which can lead to folliculitis. A thin application is all that is needed so that the skin glistens and clothing is not unduly stained.

It is important to remind parents and children of the benefits of emollients, stressing that even when the eczema is under control, it is still essential to continue the emollient therapy. Encouraging the child from as early an age as possible to apply emollients to an 'itchy bit', rather than scratch, is essential. It is also beneficial to allow the child to mess around with emollients, perhaps decorating a small container to hold some. This will familiarise the child with emollients and their importance and, in turn, encourage their application to be an accepted and normal part of daily living.

Topical steroids

These are required to control flares of eczema. There have been several years of misinformation on the use of topical steroids and their importance in the management of atopic eczema. Many parents cite thinning of the skin and stretch marks as their main concern. Many parents will understandably be alarmed at the prospect of applying topical steroids to their child knowing that they can cause skin thinning. Taking the time to find out just what knowledge the parent has of the product, and then giving them factual information to rectify any misconceptions, will help to reassure them that, correctly used, the steroid will be safe and effective in controlling eczema flares. It is also important to explain how the topical steroid functions and the different potencies available. The aim being to use the lowest potency possible to keep the eczema under control (see *Table 8.1, pp. 126–127*).

Antihistamines

This group of drugs provide symptomatic relief of pruritus. Although the itch in eczema is not histamine-mediated, the use of antihistamines may go some way to reducing self-inflicted damage through scratching (Beltrani, 1991). Some antihistamines have a sedative effect and are not recommended for day-time use when the child needs to be alert. Used at night, for short periods of time, may offer symptomatic relief and promote a restful sleep for child and family. It may be necessary to alter times of administration depending on the child's ability to rise and be alert in the morning. Topical antihistamine preparations are not recommended because of hypersensitivity problems.

Bacterial infection

Although *Staphylococcus aureus* is not part of the normal skin flora, the skin of those with eczema is often colonised with it. It is important that this pathogen is recognised, as it is responsible for most cases of infected eczema. Infection must be suspected when there is a sudden deterioration in the eczema, wet and weeping areas, marked excoriations, and sometimes painful skin. Localised areas of infection may respond to topical antibiotics, but widespread infection must be treated with systemic antibiotics (Simpson and Hannifin, 2006). A streptococcal infection will demonstrate the same set of effects, but the skin is generally erythrodermic and the child may feel unwell.

To obtain skin sensitivities, swabs should be taken prior to commencement of antibiotic therapy; although it is often beneficial to start antibiotics immediately and not wait until the swab result.

If there is infection, it is necessary to alter the general skin care regime for a short while. Antimicrobial soap substitutes and bath emollients are indicated. In cases of recurrent infections, it is advisable to re-check what treatments the child is receiving and ensure that they are being administered regularly and correctly. If the parent has reduced or discontinued use of topical steroids too soon, the itching may increase, which subsequently causes the child to scratch and so introduce infection. It is also beneficial to check staphylococcal carriage sites, such as the nasal passages of the child and parents.

Viral infections

Sufferers have an increased susceptibility to viral infections, such as *molluscum contagiosum* and herpes simplex (HS) (Hunter *et al*, 1989).

Molluscum contagiosum

Molluscum are small, flesh-coloured papules, with a central white punctum. They are generally found in the flexures but can appear anywhere and, through scratching, often become secondarily bacterially infected. The main treatment is cryotherapy, but many children will not tolerate this procedure and the molluscum can be left untreated and will generally resolve, but this can take many months. The family will need a great deal of reassurance about this.

Herpes simplex (HS)

Herpes simplex is a common infection caused by the herpes virus, hominis, of which there are two classifications:

- type 1: the cause of cold sores
- type 2: the cause of genital herpes and neonatal infections.

The virus is characterised by small clusters of vesicles on the skin surface and the buccal mucosa, which forms a crust. It generally lasts 3–6 days. Herpes simplex can cause the skin to become impetiginised.

The child with atopic eczema appears to have an abnormal response to herpes simplex, and it will rapidly disseminate to eczema herpeticum with associated toxaemia (Harper, 1990).

In this instance, the vesicles take on a punched out appearance and this condition constitutes a dermatological emergency. Treatment must be initiated promptly in the form of oral antivirals and, in more severe cases, the child will generally require hospitalisation for intravenous antiviral treatment and close observation. If any vesicles are observed on and/or around the eye, the child must immediately be referred to the ophthalmologist as there is the risk of corneal scarring.

Parents who suffer from herpes simplex should be informed of the potential risk to the child and avoid mouth to skin contact if the virus is active. Staff who have an active cold sore should not have contact with a child suffering from eczema.

Nutrition

To gain an insight into dietary status, it is important to gather the following information on your initial contact with the child. The child's height and weight will be recorded in patient records, check if they are within normal limit — it is useful to plot them on a growth chart. Establish if the child is on any form of exclusion diet and, if so, try and get the rationale for parental decision and record who is monitoring, supervising and supporting the parent in this? Many parents find it difficult to accept that there is no cure for this condition, and are often in receipt of confusing and conflicting information on causes of eczema and many are led to believe that food, especially milk, is the cause. A trial of dietary manipulation is only indicated when the child's history is strongly suggestive of a specific food allergy, or where there is widespread active eczema failing to respond to first-line therapy. Atopic eczema is triggered by many factors. Few pathogenic aspects are accepted as fact. The disease is strongly familial, multigenic with genetic associations to allergic rhinitis, asthma and atopy (Simpson and Hanifin, 2006). Although approximately 30% of sufferers may have food allergy as a trigger, and for 10% of these it will be the main trigger, it is rare for diet to be the cause for atopic eczema (National Eczema Society [NES], 2003).

Whether or not food allergy is suspected, after medical history it is essential that the initial visit should focus on skin care. The parents must be given adequate information on the importance of fundamental skin care, and encouraged to focus on this rather than on dietary exclusions (Simpson and Hanifin, 2006)

It will be necessary to refer the child to the dietician to support and educate the parent as well as assess if the child is having adequate nutritional intake (McHenry, 1995). Some skin disorders may be triggered by or manifest from inadequate nutrition.

If it is reported that the child is 'allergic to something', ask the parents to describe exactly what happened during the incident and what action was initiated. It is important to discover if it is a true allergy and if any investigations have already been undertaken, and the outcome of any results. RAST (radioallergosorbent test) may be helpful in planning the management of the child; it identifies the total IgE level and specific allergens, such as food and pollens.

Nursery/school

Parents should be encouraged to discuss the child's eczema with nursery/school prior to the beginning of term. It is essential that the nursery/school have as much information as possible to enable the child to be comfortable and to mix and join in with peers. Teachers/leaders must be aware that eczema is erratic and varies in severity and can be constantly changing.

Children should have the majority of treatment carried out in the home, but it will often be necessary for emollients to be applied during the nursery/school day. At school, the application of emollients should be carried out during a structured break time and not be allowed to disrupt the lesson. It is a good idea to remember the need for a soap substitute, as regular contact with soap will undoubtedly irritate the child's skin.

There are several environmental factors that can minimise discomfort in the nursery/school, such as seating the child away from heaters and sunny windows.

The regular use of sedating antihistamines can have a residual knock-on effect, and may result in the child being drowsy in the class. This should be observed and the timing of administration altered if necessary.

It is unreasonable to expect the child with eczema not to scratch, and constantly telling the child not to do so will be upsetting and possibly cause unnecessary stress. In the event of a scratching frenzy, it is worth trying to distract the child. However, if this disrupts the other children, the child should be temporarily removed to try and calm him/her down through the application of emollients.

Acceptance by peers is crucial to all children's development but school, in particular, can cause a great deal of stress and anxiety for children with eczema. They may lose valuable education through frequent absences, and these absences can also lead to exclusion by peers. There is the potential for the child to be ridiculed and bullied because of the appearance of their skin. They may be unable to take part in some sport and hobbies because of their eczema. Teachers need to observe for any signs of unhappiness and discuss with the parents and child as necessary.

The National Eczema Society produce excellent guidelines for schools. Encourage parents to make this clear to the nursery/school and, indeed, to obtain them and pass them on to relevant school personnel.

Effect on family

Caring for the child with eczema has the potential to impose an enormous psychological burden on a family who will consequently require a great deal of support.

The main carer of the child may find it exhausting and, despite putting in a great deal of time and effort, there is often little reward. Treatments tend to be time-consuming and monotonous — motivation is crucial. It is important both to recognise and discuss this with the carer, in order to support them and encourage them to develop a consistent skin care regime that fits in with family life, as far as possible. This can prove difficult during times when little or no improvement in the child's eczema is perceived. Additional support may be indicated when the child rebels against the skin care.

Tools designed for children with skin problems, such as the Children's Dermatology Life Quality Index (CDLQI; Lewis-Jones and Finlay, 1995), and the Infant's Dermatitis Quality of Life Index (IDQLI), will help to assess the impact of eczema on a family.

A study by Lawson _et al_ (1998), using the Dermatology Life Quality Index (DLQI) and the CDLQI, examined the impact on the family of having a child with atopic eczema, and gives an excellent insight into the effect of caring for the child. It identified the following:

* 74% of parents described the burden of household cleaning and laundry, and the preparation of food.
* 71% of parents described psychological pressures, guilt, exhaustion, frustration, resentment and helplessness.
* 66% of parents said that they did not have a normal family life, identifying restrictions around pets, laundry products and food.

* 63% of children have sleep problems and many have sleep disturbances. Itching and scratching lead to exhaustion and frustration in 64% of parents, and sleep disturbances in 63%.
* Six out of ten school-aged children experienced teasing and bullying.
* 54% of parents identified behaviour problems in the child, such as being irritable, naughty, bad-tempered and easily bored.
* 34% of parents felt that they had a limited social life due to tiredness; locating a suitable babysitter was also identified.
* 29% of parents felt that interpersonal relationships were adversely affected and identified sleep loss as a source of friction. Some identified being overprotective to the child, leading to family resentment.
* 17% of parents felt that they did not receive adequate support from teaching and medical professionals .
* 23% of families had holiday restrictions because of sleeping problems, climate change, and special requirements for creams, clothing and bedding.

This study also identified financial issues, ie. extra costs for clothing, linen and food.

Practical help when caring for a child with eczema

There are several factors known to aggravate eczema and these should be avoided as far as possible, namely:

* Avoid extremes of temperature, this is particularly important to consider when carrying out a bathing regime.
* Keeping the child's fingernails short will help to minimise damage through scratching.
* Biological detergents and fabric softeners should be avoided as they will irritate the skin.

Clothing

Factors to consider with regard to clothing, include:

❖ All-in-one, cotton sleep-suits which button up at the back will minimise damage to the skin through scratching at night. They can also be worn during the day if not in school.
❖ Try and encourage use of cotton clothing and linen, which is more comfortable to the child. Wool will irritate the skin.
❖ Cotton gloves can be worn in bed and also for activities such as painting.

House dust mites

It is the droppings, not the actual parasite, that causes irritation to the eczematous skin. Although it is not possible to eradicate them completely from a house, it is possible to adopt some practices that will reduce their activity, such as by:

❖ Keeping the sleeping area cool and well-ventilated as house dust mites prefer warm, humid environments.
❖ Encouraging the use of anti house dust mite protector covers for all mattresses and pillows, and using cotton bed linen. If the child sleeps in a bunk bed, he/she should ideally sleep on the top bunk.
❖ Damp-dusting bedrooms and vacuuming carpets regularly; uncarpeted environments are preferable for the child.
❖ Washing bed linen at a high temperature of 60°C. This will kill the mites.
❖ Placing favourite toys in the freezer overnight and washing them, as toys also hoard house dust mites.

To control the symptoms of eczema, it is crucial that parents and, where appropriate, the child, understand how and when to use treatments, and the importance of using them. All verbal information should be supplemented with written information. Ensure that the family have contact details of those who can support them, advising them of support networks.

It may be necessary to initiate more complex treatment strategies if the eczema cannot be controlled by first-line measures: these should, however, be carried out under specialist supervision. It is crucial that healthcare professionals caring for the child with eczema are aware that this is not just a trivial skin disorder, but a condition that will need continuous, ongoing support.

References

Beltrani V (1999) Managing atopic eczema. *Dermatol Nurs* **11**(3): 171–85

Bridgett C, Noren P, Staughton R (1996) *Atopic Skin Disease: A manual for practitioners.* Wrightson Biomedical Publishing Ltd, USA

Brown S, Reynolds NJ (2006) Atopic and non-atopic eczema. *Br Med J* **332**(7541): 584–8

Cork M (1997) The importance of skin barrier function. *J Dermatological Treatments* (supplement) **8**(1): 7–13

Harper J (1990) *Handbook of Paediatric Dermatology.* 2nd edn. Butterworth-Heinemann, London

Hoare C, Po A, Williams HH (2000) Systematic reveiw of treatments for atopic eczema. *Health Technol Assess* **4**(37): 1–191

Hunter JAA, Savin JA, Dahl MV (1989) *Clinical Dermatology.* Blackwell Scientific Publications, Oxford, chap 15: 150–4

Lewis-Jones MS, Finlay AY (1995) The Children's Dermatology Life Quality Index (CDLQI). Initial validation and practical use. *Br J Dermatol* **132**: 942–9

McHenry PM, Williams HC, Bingham EA (1995) Management of atopic eczema. Joint workshop of the British Association of Dermatologists and the Research Unit of the Royal College of Physicians of London. *Br Med J* **310**(6983): 843–7

National Eczema Society (2003) *Diet and eczema in children.* NES, London

Lawson V, Lewis-Jones MS, Finlay AY, Reid P, Owens RG (1998) The family impact of childhood atopic dermatitis: The Dermatitis Family Impact Questionnaire. *Br J Dermatol* **138**(1): 107–13

Robinson J (2003) Atopic eczema. In: Barnes K, ed. *Paediatrics: a clinical guide for nurse practitioners.* Butterworth-Heinemann, Edinburgh

Simpson EL, Hanifin JM (2006) Atopic dermatitis. *Med Clin N Am* **90**: 149–67

Recommended reading and useful websites

Cork MJ (1998) _Complete Emollient Therapy. The National Association of Fundholding Practices Official Yearbook._ BPC Waterlow, Dunstable: 159–68

Gawkrodger D (2003) _Dermatology. An illustrated colour text._ 3rd edn. Churchill Livingstone, Edinburgh

Hanifin JM, Cooper KD, Ho VC _et al_ (2004) Guidelines of care for atopic dermatitis. _J Am Acad Dermatol_ **50**(3): 391–404

Holden C, English J _et al_ (2002) Advised Best Practice for the use of emollients in eczema and other dry skin conditions. _J Dermatological Treatments_ **13**: 103–6

Hughes E, Van Onselen (2001) _Dermatology Nursing: A practical guide._ Churchill Livingstone, Edinburgh

Turnbull R (2003) Management of atopic eczema in children. _J Community Nurs_ **7**(6): 32–6

British Association of Dermatologists, available online at:www.bad.org.uk/public/leaflets

British Skin Foundation, available online at: www.britishskinfoundation.org.uk

National Eczema Society, available online at: www.eczema.org

National Guideline Clearinghouse, available online at: www.guideline.gov

	Mild	Moderate	Potent	Very potent	Formulation
Table: 8.1: Comparison of the therapeutic potencies and formulations of topical steroids					

Table: 8.1: Comparison of the therapeutic potencies and formulations of topical steroids

Potency

	Mild	Moderate	Potent	Very potent	Formulation
Acorvio Plus*			●		Cream
Alphaderm*		●			Cream
Alphosyl HC*	●				Cream
Aureocort*			●		Ointment
Betacap			●		Scalp application
Betnovate			●		Cream, ointment, lotion, scalp application
Betnovate RD		●			Cream, ointment
Betnovate C*			●		Cream, ointment
Betnovate N*			●		Cream, ointment
Bettamousse			●		Scalp application
Calmurid HC*		●			Cream
Canesten HC*	●				Cream
Clarelux				●	Scalp application
Cutivate			●		Cream, ointment
Daktacort*	●				Cream, ointment
Dermovate				●	Cream, ointment, scalp application
Dermovate NN*				●	Cream
Dioderm	●				Cream
Diprosalic*			●		Ointment, scalp application
Diprosone			●		Cream, ointment, lotion
Dovobet*			●		Ointment
Econacort*	●				Cream
Efcortelan	●				Cream, ointment
Elocon			●		Cream, ointment, scalp application
Eumovate		●			Cream, ointment
Eurax-Hydrocortisone*	●				Cream
Fucibet*			●		Cream
Fucidin H*	●				Cream, ointment
Haelan		●			Cream, ointment, tape
Halciderm				●	Cream

Table: 8.1: Cont.

	Mild	Moderate	Potent	Very potent	Formulation
Potency					
Locoid			●		Cream, emulsion, ointment, oily cream, scalp application
Locoid C*			●		Cream, ointment
Lotriderm*			●		Cream
Metosyn			●		Cream, ointment
Mildison Lipocream	●				Oily cream
Modrasone		●			Cream, ointment
Nerisone			●		Cream, ointment, oily cream
Nerisone Forte				●	Ointment, oily cream
Nystaform HC*	●				Cream, ointment
Propaderm			●		Ointment
Synalar			●		Cream, ointment, gel (for scalp application)
Synalar 1:4		●			Cream, ointment
Synalar 1:10	●				Cream
Synalar C*			●		Cream, ointment
Synalar N*			●		Cream, ointment
Timodine*	●				Cream
Tri-Adcortyl*			●		Cream, ointment
Trimovate*		●			Cream
Ultralanum*		●			Cream, ointment
Vioform-Hydrocortisone*	●				Cream, ointment

Reproduced by kind permission of MIMS Haymarket Publishing

* = product has at least one other active ingredient
Severity of side-effects is related to various factors, in addition, therapeutic potency and the two are, therefore, not necessarily interrelated, particularly where skin is damaged

Table 8.2: Moisturisers, potential skin sensitisers as ingredients

	Fragrances	Beeswax	Cetyl/Cetostearyl/Stearyl alcohol	Propylene glycol	Triethanolamine	Lanolin/derivatives	Benzalkonium chloride	Benzyl alcohol	Hydroxybenzoates (parabens)	Phenethyl alcohol	Phenoxyethanol	Quarternium-15	Sorbic acid/sorbates	Triclosan	Butylated hydroxyanisole	Butylated hydroxytoluene	Other potential sensitisers
Alpha keri	●					●											❶
Aquadrate																	
Aveeno bath additive																	
Aveeno bath oil	●	●												●			
Aveeno cream			●					●									
Balneum bath oil	●			●												●	
Balneum plus cream								●									
Balneum plus oil	●			●												●	
Calmurid																	
Cetraben emollient bath additive																	
Cetraben emollient cream			●						●		●						
Dermalo bath emollient						●											
Dermamist																	
Dermol 200 shower emollient			●				●				●						❷
Dermol 500 lotion			●				●				●						
Dermol 600 bath emollient							●						●				

Table 8.2: Cont.

	Fragrances	Beeswax	Cetyl/Cetostearyl/Stearyl alcohol	Propylene glycol	Triethanolamine	Lanolin/derivatives	Benzalkonium chloride	Benzyl alcohol	Hydroxybenzoates (parabens)	Phenethyl alcohol	Phenoxyethanol	Quarternium-15	Sorbic acid/sorbates	Triclosan	Butylated hydroxyanisole	Butylated hydroxytoluene	Other potential sensitisers
Dermol cream							•										❷
Diprobase cream			•														❸
Diprobase ointment																	
Diprobath																	
Doublebase				•							•						
E45 bath oil																	
E45 cream			•			•			•								
E45 lotion						•		•	•								
E45 wash cream																	
Emulsiderm							•						•				
Epaderm			•														
Eucerin						•		•									
Eumobase		•	•														
Eurax cream	•	•	•		•				•	•							❹
Eurax lotion	•		•	•							•			•			❹
Gamma-derm		•	•	•					•		•		•				
Hydromol cream			•						•		•						
Hydromol emollient																	
Hydromol ointment																	
Imuderm	•														•		

Table 8.2: Cont.

	Fragrances	Beeswax	Cetyl/Cetostearyl/Stearyl alcohol	Propylene glycol	Triethanolamine	Lanolin/derivatives	Benzalkonium chloride	Benzyl alcohol	Hydroxybenzoates (parabens)	Phenethyl alcohol	Phenoxyethanol	Quarternium-15	Sorbic acid/sorbates	Triclosan	Butylated hydroxyanisole	Butylated hydroxytoluene	Other potential sensitisers
Infaderm	•													•			
Kamillosan		•				•			•								❺
Keri	•			•	•	•			•			•					
Lipobase			•						•								
Morhulin						•											
Nutraplus				•					•								
Oilatum cream			•	•				•					•				
Oilatum emollient	•					•											
Oilatum emollient fragrant free						•											
Oilatum gel	•																
Oilatum junior cream			•					•					•				
Oilatum plus						•	•							•			
Sprilon			•			•											
Sudocrem	•	•		•		•		•							•		*
Ultrabase cream	•		•						•								**
Unguentum M			•	•									•				
Vasogen						•					•						
Xepin			•					•									
Zerobase			•														❸

Reproduced by kind permission of MIMS, Haymarket Publishing

* Benzyl benzoate, benzykl cinnamate, ** Disodium edetate, ❶ Oxybenzone, ❷ Chlorhexidine, ❸ Chlorocresol, ❹ Crotamiton, ❺ Camomile extract

Appendix

1. Was pregnancy normal?

2. Was the baby born at full term? Was it a normal delivery?

3. Was the skin normal at birth

4. Was the baby breast fed? Until what age? Weaned onto what formula?

5. At what age did the eczema start?

   - Where on the body did it start
   - Further details about eczema (eg. hours of sleep disturbance)

6. What treatment have you had so far (including frequency of baths)?

7. Has your child had much time off school because of the eczema?

   - Does eczema stop your child from doing anything?

8. Does the sun make the eczema worse or better?

9. Have you changed the baby's diet?

10. Do you have pets, or does the child have contact with pets at any time?

11. Details about bedding, toys, etc.

12. Has infection of the skin been a problem?

13. Is your child prone to infections of the chest/ear, etc?

14. Has your child all vaccinations to date?

15. Is there a family history of eczema, asthma or hayfever?

16. Are there any smokers around the child?

17. How do you wash the baby's clothes? Are they cotton as far as possible?

18. Does your child have asthma?

19. Has your child ever had an allergic reaction?

20. Has your child ever had urticaria?

This appendix is reproduced courtesy of Dr Nerys Roberts, Consultant Dermatologist, Chelsea and Westminster Hospital, London

CHAPTER 9

PAEDIATRIC STOMA CARE

Pat Coldicutt

The first record of a successfully performed colostomy on an infant was by Duret in 1798 on a four-day-old infant with anorectal agenesis (Dinnick, 1934; Parry, 1998). In the early 1940s, a small group of patients in the USA formed a self-help group, which developed into the United Ostomy Associations of America (UOAA) in the 1950s (Johnson, 1992). In 1956, the first European support group was conceived and became the Ileostomy Association of Great Britain. In subsequent years, the Urostomy Support Group was set up and, as late as 1985, the children's support group called the National Advisory Service to Parents of Children with a Stoma (NASPCS) led by parents for parents was established (Johnson, 1992). From these groups it was identified that further help and support was required, and in the early 1970s, the first stoma care nurse was appointed and the first stoma care nursing course evolved. Throughout the UK today, there are approximately 350 stoma care nurses, and in every paediatric centre a stoma nurse post exists. As paediatric stoma care nurses we are in a privileged position caring for vulnerable infants, children and young people. All these families and children need to be treated in a delicate and sensitive manner. It is crucial that they are given the support and are empowered to carry out their child's care (Kennedy, 1992).

There are a number of reasons for stoma formation in children. Regional centres across the UK perform between 100–200 stomas per year, and the majority of them are temporary stomas, which are often reversed after a few months following corrective surgery. Eighty percent of paediatric stoma surgery takes place during the first six weeks of life, 10% from six weeks to one year, and the remaining 10%

are performed in older children with inflammatory bowel disease or trauma (Fitzpatrick, 2001).

Congenital abnormalities

Imperforate anus

Anorectal abnormalities occur 1 in every 5000 live births; they are known as imperforate anus and can be divided into three groups (Black, 2000). Low imperforate anus occurs when the rectal pouch ends blindly — anal agenesis. Treatment involves opening or moving the anus, thus making a connection, and is known as an anoplasty which can be performed at birth. These infants have a good prognosis. High defects occur above the pelvic floor musculature and require extensive surgery (Peria, 1994). The bowel ends in a blind pouch or continuous fistula. In boys, it is known as rectourethral fistula and, in girls, rectovaginal fistula. These infants require a colostomy and further surgery (Fitzpatrick, 2001). The third group, intermediate imperforate anus, occurs between the other two groups.

Hirschsprung's disease

Hirschsprung's disease is a genetic disorder which was named by Harold Hirschsprung, the Dutch physician, who first described the disease in 1886 after caring for two boys who were unable to have spontaneous bowel movements. Hirschsprung's disease is caused by the absence of nerve cells in the wall of the bowel.

Collections of nerve cells, or ganglia, control the co-ordinated relaxation of the bowel wall that is necessary for bowel contents to advance. Failure of this process to occur results in constipation. Babies born with Hirschsprung's disease often have difficulty passing meconuim. This affects one baby in every 5000 live births, and often they present with abdominal distention, and bile-stained vomiting. Diagnosis is achieved by rectal biopsy, either suction or full thickness (Johnson, 1992). The treatment includes surgery to remove the affected bowel and then to join the healthy segments. The surgery can be carried out in one stage, where the affected segment is removed and the healthy bowel brought down into the rectum (pull through). Sometimes a colostomy is fashioned and the pull through is done at a later stage (Roback, 1988). The surgery often depends on the health of the child and the surgeon's preference.

Necrolising enterocolitis (NEC)

This is largely a disease of pre-term infants, characterised by one or more areas of intestinal necrosis interspersed with segments of normal bowel being affected. The terminal ileum, right colon, left colon and sigmoid colon are the most commonly involved sites (Pokorny _et al_, 1995). Infants with NEC are usually managed medically with complete bowel rest, intravenous fluids, nasogastric decompression and antibiotics (Rogers, 2003). Surgical intervention is indicated when the infant fails to respond to medical treatment, or if gangrene or perforation of the bowel occurs. Twenty-five to fifty percent of newborns with NEC require surgery (Caty _et al_, 2000).

Meconium ileus

Meconium ileus results from abnormalities of exocrine mucus secretion, which contributes to the production of thick, sticky meconium that obstructs the small intestinal lumen. Ninety-five percent of infants who have meconium ileus will have cystic fibrosis (Haga, 1999). Obstruction usually occurs in the distal 15–30 cms of terminal ileum. Surgery may be required, with the formation of an end-to-end anastomosis of the bowel to relieve the obstruction, followed by fashioning of an ileostomy.

Inflammatory bowel diseases

Inflammatory bowel diseases, such as Crohn's disease and ulcerative colitis, are rare in children. They are often successfully managed medically and only a small percentage require surgery. Crohn's disease is an inflammation of the gastrointestinal tract, and can start in the mouth and go all the way through to the rectum. The inflammation goes through the bowel wall and is not just limited to the mucosal lining (Williams and Nichols, undated). Due to advancement in medical treatment, these patients can be managed effectively; however, if the patient is suspected of having bowel perforation, surgery is crucial. Ulcerative colitis, which affects the colon, is rare in children. It can be treated medically with anti-inflammatory drugs, enemas and, occasionally, steroid therapy.

Preparation of the patient (infant)

As previously stated, the majority of patients who require stoma formations are infants born with congenital abnormalities, and so it can be difficult to assess these infants and their families prior to surgery. However, when possible, it is advised to discuss the issues with the infant's parents. It must be remembered that the parents have dreamt about their expectations of their child, and are devastated when they are told that their long-awaited infant faces surgery. A sensitive, sympathetic approach should be adopted to gain their trust and to assist them through a difficult time.

Before surgery the patient's history should be taken, including whether the patient has asthma, eczema, any other skin conditions, or any allergies. It may be necessary to carry out patch testing with the various flanges to ensure that the patient does not have any allergy to the particular product. This involves placing small pieces of each flange on various places of the abdomen to ascertain if the patient has any reaction. The parents are instructed to number each flange piece and to keep a record to ensure that, if any reaction does occur, this product can be avoided .

Assessment

The first consideration after stabilisation of the infant's condition is the stoma site. In the neonate, the surgery is often emergent, with no time for assessment of the abdomen. In addition, depending on the infant's condition, the abdomen may be distorted because of the disease process, eg. obstruction. It is also difficult, if not impossible, to predict physical growth in a baby, therefore, selection of the stoma site is rarely done (Boarini, 1989). There are several factors that a paediatric surgeon should consider when creating a stoma for an infant. The stoma should be positioned away from the umbilicus, allowing space for the adhesive to be placed and, when the cord has fallen off, preventing an uneven surface for the pouch to stick on to. The stoma should not be placed too low on the abdominal wall, as babies wriggle in ways that an adult cannot. The pouch can be difficult to apply if the infant brings his legs up and the site is near the groin. Good positioning of the stoma prevents problems, such as sore skin and leakage.

As the infant improves and recovers from surgery, the parents are empowered to care for their baby and are taught how to clean the delicate skin, cut and apply the pouch correctly. Continual assessment of the family is required to enable the nurses to assess the level of the family's coping mechanisms, and how much support and intervention they require throughout their child's hospital stay.

Assessment of the older child

Before admission for ostomy surgery, it is important to meet the child/young person, preferably in their own environment. Generally, the family have been given the news by the surgeon in clinic and the forthcoming surgery will have been discussed. The stoma care nurse should start the preparation by assessing the child's/young person's comprehension of what they already know.

It is important to explain in a language that they understand, and allow any questions to be asked and answered honestly. Throughout this meeting, the stoma nurse will be noting their likes and dislikes, social activity, manual dexterity, and their acceptance of the illness. She/he will also be observing the interaction between the parents and the child/young person.

Stoma sites

The stoma site should be marked pre-operatively, avoiding any bony prominences, scars, the waistline and groin, and marking the correct side, depending on the type of stoma surgery to be performed. This should be carried out with both the child/young person's consent and with the parents present. Where possible, document the site of the mark and get the parents to sign that they were present and witnessed the mark being made.

Pouch selection

There are many types of stoma appliances, however, the range is somewhat limited for children. The type of pouch chosen will depend on the type of stoma the child/young person has. The choice for infants is often a one-piece, drainable pouch, which allows the faeces to be drained and the pouch can remain in place on an infant's delicate abdomen for a number of days. This will be selected for children with both a colostomy and an ileostomy. The family are taught how to drain the faeces out, although with a colostomy this can be difficult. The parents are advised to add a small amount of baby oil to the bag to help the faeces glide out easily. The older child/young person will choose the pouch themselves, after being shown a range of different ones. They usually choose a two-piece system, drainable for the ileostomist and closed for the colostomist. Children prefer the two-piece systems as they can be removed quickly and easily, and can be discarded without having to remove the adhesive flange, for example, when going out with friends, attending school, or swimming. This also allows for the smaller pouch to be used in conjunction with the same adhesive flange.

Skin care/protection

The best type of skin care is prevention. This is why it is crucial to position the stoma correctly, thus preventing problems from occurring.

Following surgery, infants are normally nursed without a pouch for the first 24–48 hours, until the stoma is active. The pouch of choice is usually a one-piece, clear drainable one, which allows the nurse to observe the colour of the stoma without disturbing the pouch. Pouches are available in a range of sizes, from those which have a starter hole to enable easy cutting of the pouch, to those without a starter hole. The latter type is particularly helpful for pre-term infants whose stoma is smaller than the usual 8mm starter hole size, or for awkwardly placed stomas that require a smaller pouch. Pelican have introduced both a neonatal and paediatric pouch with a teddy bear design on it. They have a split-back section which allows easy vision when applying the pouch, but covers the stoma afterwards, thus preventing the output from being observed which some parents prefer. ConvaTec also have a clear, drainable pouch which has a larger flange area. This is helpful for infants that have a divided colostomy, and allows both stomas to be incorporated in the bag if they are positioned close together. Drainable, one-piece pouches are generally used for infants with either a colostomy or an ileostomy. If the faeces are of a thick consistency, the pouch can be lightly coated with baby oil prior to application, which allows the thick faeces to slide out and assists drainage.

Once the pouch has been selected it remains *in situ* for 3–4 days. This prevents the peri-stomal skin becoming sore, and preserves the skin's integrity. Parents are advised to remove the pouch if it needs changing, ie. if it has started to leak or redness is observed. This is done by gently soaking around the adhesive part of the pouch with warm water and removing it from the top downwards. Warm water and unperfumed soap are recommended. This can also be done while the infant is in the bath. Adhesive removers impregnated with an orange oil are also available. These can easily be applied to the adhesive area on the flange, lifting the flange away without pain or trauma. They should not be used if the patient is allergic to oranges. The skin should be cleansed afterwards in warm, soapy water to remove the oily residue left. Correct cutting of the flange prevents sore skin and assists with adhesion of the pouch. Gently warming the pouch prior to use also helps to activate the adhesive properties. The use of pastes is rarely advised, as some contain alcohol and sting, and others tend to be difficult to remove and, if used incorrectly, can cause trauma and skin breakdown.

Skin protection should not be required; however, there are a range of products available within stoma care.

Cavilon™ Spray and Applicator (3M™)

This product can be applied directly onto sore, red skin without stinging. It must be used with care, and the stoma should be covered to prevent occlusion from the spray. The spray is easy to direct and can be used on large areas of soreness. It should be applied according to the manufacturer's guidance.

Skin protector wipes

These come in sachets and can easily be carried in your bag. They can be used directly on sore skin and are single use only, reducing the risk of infection. They create a protective film which prevents the faecal enzymes burning the peri-stomal skin. For patients with an allergy, these can also be applied to the skin prior to application of the flange.

Protective wafers

These are particularly helpful for patients who have any creases, dips, or contours on their abdomen that require building up. The wafers can be applied to level out the contours, creating a smooth surface before the pouch is applied.

Washers, strip paste

These are ideal for the hard-to-reach areas. If the patient has a dip or crease between the suture line or stoma, a small piece of washer or strip paste can be moulded and applied to the problem area. They can also be used if a specific area of the flange is not sticking. A small piece can be warmed and moulded and applied to the back of the flange before application, and then placed over the problem area.

Possible problems following stoma surgery

Skin breakdown

Adaptation to life with a stoma depends to a large extent on the health of the peri-stomal skin (Black, 2000). Skin problems are the major complications facing nurses responsible for stoma care. The skin of the pre-term infant is at risk of breakdown from pouch adhesives because it lacks full tensile strength. Therefore, it is essential that the correct selection of pouch adhesive is made.

Flush stoma

This is where the stoma mucosa is at a level with the skin, either circumferential or partially. A stoma may be flush because of surgical technique difficulties, eg. poor mobilisation of the bowel, or due to excess weight gain. The problems that are likely to occur include obtaining and maintaining a secure, leak-proof seal. This is particularly the case in the management of an ileostomy due to the liquid nature of the output. The solution is to select a suitable appliance; a convexity product is often the one of choice.

Mucocutaneous separation — infection

This occurs because of a breakdown in the suture line, between the bowel mucosa and the skin securing the stoma to the abdominal surface. This has occurred in neonates between the stoma and the mucus fistula. Treatment involves application of a ribbon Hydrofiber® dressing (Aquacel®, ConvaTec) over the affected area, with a hydrocolloid dressing to keep it in position (*Figure 9.1*). The pouch is then cut to size and placed over the stoma. The Hydrofiber® dressing is made of 100% carboxymethylcellulose polymer. The hydrophilic action allows rapid absorption of exudate which is retained in the Hydrofiber®. Removal is usually painless and skin-friendly (Williams,

1999). It requires changing every 2–3 days; if the pouch leaks, more frequent changes are needed.

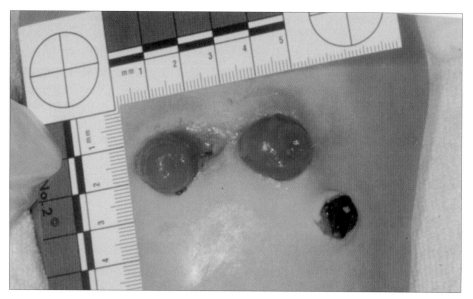

Figure 9.1: Infant with a transverse divided colostomy, showing infected suture line. Treated by gentle cleaning with warm Normasol® (Mölnlycke Health Care), applying Aquacel® (ConvaTec) to the infected area and covering this with DuoDERM® (ConvaTec). A clear, drainable pouch was then cut to size and placed over the top

Contact dermatitis

This is when the patient suffers an allergic reaction to the appliance. This normally occurs where the adhesive touches the abdomen but, in extreme cases, may occur where the plastic of the appliance touches the abdomen. Contact dermatitis has a geometric outline that follows the shape of the adhesive area. This is known as picture framing. Patients will often have a previous history of sensitivity reactions, which should have been elucidated pre-operatively. In extreme cases of known sensitivity, it is advised to carry out pre-operative patch testing. Contact dermatitis may be resolved by changing to another appliance. Most appliances are hypoallergenic and contact dermatitis is less frequent (Lyon and Beck, 2001).

Red, sore skin and leakage

This is due to an ill-fitting appliance (*Figure 9.2*). The flange is cut too large and the peri-stomal skin comes into contact with the faecal output. This results in leakage under the flange. Once removed, the flange should be flipped over to ascertain the problem area. Particular attention should be given to this area to ensure that the flange has been correctly cut when it is being re-applied. The peri-stomal skin should be washed gently with unperfumed soap and warm water. Often, a light dusting of Orahesive powder is effective when treating moist, raw areas, but too much will prevent the adhesive sticking. Nurses may worry that placing an appliance on red skin will make it worse, so they need reassurance that this is not the case. Gently cleansing and patting dry the skin, and applying a new, correctly cut flange, will assist the skin healing process. If left in place for 3–4 days, an improvement is usually noted after removal. Creams cannot be used as they also affect the adhesive properties of appliances (Webster, 1985). If the patient has an ileostomy, the output is often watery. Problems can occur due to the weight of the fluid output. Frequent emptying of the pouch is advised via a drainable pouch. Absorbent sachets, or gels, can be added to solidify the output. Infant fluid output should be carefully monitored to prevent excessive fluid and salt loss. This can cause dehydration and extra fluids and salt supplements should be given.

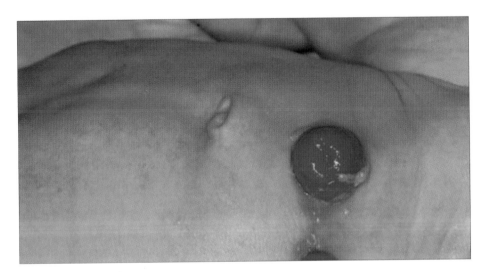

Figure 9.2: Redness and soreness

Allergies

An allergy can occur with any substance that comes into contact with an infant's skin (*Figure 9.3*). If this is the case, the infant is sometimes nursed without a pouch and the peri-stomal skin is protected by soft paraffin and/or protective skin products, such as Cavilon™ applicator. Gauze is also used and removed as soon as it becomes soiled.

If allergies are a problem for the older child or young person, it is important to remove the products that the patient is allergic to and try other types. The nurse should keep close observation of the patient and persist with each appliance. This is why patch testing is so important if allergy is suspected prior to surgery.

Retraction

Stoma retraction occurs when the child gains weight, or if there is insufficient bowel used to construct the stoma in the first place (Hagelgans and Janusz, 1994). The treatment is usually resolved with further surgery; the stoma is often reversed in these cases. If this is not possible, the use of convexity products are recommended. Convexity is defined as the outward curving of the flange or skin barrier. The convexity allows for continuous contact and creates pressure on the peri-stomal area to partly evert the retracted stoma (Dansac). It can be assisted further by wearing a belt connected to the flange at each side. Care should be taken as this type of flange can create pressure ulcers.

Prolapse

This is the protrusion of the stoma through abdominal musculature (Hagelgans and Janusz, 1994). Often the stoma will prolapse without warning, or following a bout of coughing or crying. If patients and their families are aware of the risk, it will be less of a shock in the event of it happening. Warm saline soaks help to reduce the problem, but may not solve it. Even with some warning, it can be extremely frightening for the parents. If the stoma remains pink and active, surgery is often not performed. Sometimes a larger pouch is required to accommodate the increase in size and length of the patient's stoma.

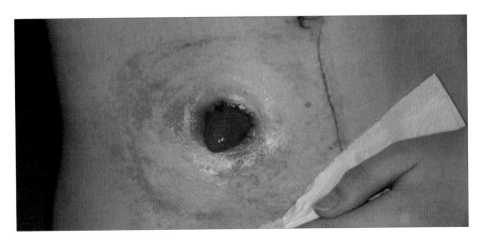

Figure 9.3: Candida infection and allergy to adhesive tape

Candidiasis (moniliasis)

Candidiasis is a cutaneous or mucosal infection caused by the yeast *Candida albicans*. Stoma patients are susceptible to candida infection because the peri-stomal area is warm and moist. Treatment consists of prescribed antifungal medications, such as miconazole or clotrimazole, the latter is available in spray form and is useful for treating peri-stomal rashes (*Figure 9.4*).

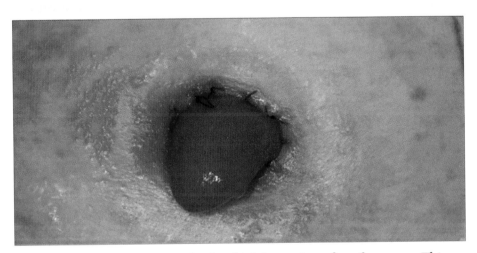

Figure 9.4: A young person who has had formation of an ileostomy. This shows candida infection which is treated by topical antifungal preparations. Powders are preferable to creams as they allow adhesion of the flange

Discharge

Once the child/young person/parents have mastered the stoma care management they are able to go home. The families will have continued support by either a paediatric community nurse, stoma nurse, or a district nurse. They are informed of the patient's discharge details and arrangements for follow-up between the family and the nurse. This allows on-going care and support in the community for as long as it is required. The family's general practitioner is also contacted to update them on the child's condition, and will supply all the products needed for the patient's stoma care at home (Jefferies *et al*, 1995).

Conclusion

Paediatric nurses are in a privileged position, as they are caring on a daily basis with vulnerable infants and children. They also have a responsibility to educate the parents/carers to enable them to care for their child's ostomy, given the stresses and challenges they face. Within a short period of time the parents, carers, and sometimes the children themselves, master the techniques required. Adapting to this challenge is never easy, no matter at what point in life it occurs. The infant with a congenital disorder with an ostomy faces extra challenges but, with accurate information, care and reassurance, these can be addressed.

When choosing the right appliance for children and young people, it must be remembered that each is an individual with different needs, whose best interests must be paramount (Fitzpatrick, 2001). Given the right information, problems can be kept to a minimum.

References

Black PK (1994) Common problems following stoma surgery. *Br J Nurs* 3(8): 413–7

Black PK (2000) *Holistic Stoma Care*. Baillière Tindall, Edinburgh, London: chap 18

Boarini JH (1989) Principles of stoma care for infants. _J Enterostomal Ther_ 16(1): 21–5

Caty M, Azizkhan R (2000) Necrotising enterocolitis. In: Ashcraft W, ed. _Pediatric Surgery_. 3rd edn. WB Saunders, Philadelphia: 443–52

Dinnick T (1934) The origins and evolutions of colostomy. _Br J Surg_ 22: 142–54

Fitzpatrick G (2001) Choosing the right appliance for paediatric stoma. _Nurse Prescriber/Br J Community Nurs_ June 2001: 36–7

Haga LJ (1999) Neonatal intestinal obstruction, part II. _Suturline_ 7: 1–4

Hagelgans NA, Janusz HB (1994) Paediatric skin care issues for the home care nurse, part 2. _Paediatr Nurs_ 20(1): 69–75

Hancock J (2000) Nursing the pre-term surgical neonate. _J Child Health Care_ 4(1): 12–18

Jefferies E, Joels J, Butler M, Callum R, Little G, Johnson A (1995) A service evaluation of stoma care nurses practice. _J Clin Nurs_ 4: 235–42

Johnson H (1992) Stoma care for infants and young children. _Paediatr Nurs_ 4: 8–11

Kennedy J (1992) Teaching parents to care for their infant's colostomy. _C.A.E.T J_ 16(4): 7–10

Oren M (2003) Prepare parents and child before ostomy surgery: STOMA acronym helps to reinforce steps. _Patient Education Management, Focus on Pediatrics_, August: 1–2

Parry A (1998) Stoma care in neonates— improving practice. _J Neonatal Nurs_ 4 January: 8–11

Peria A (1994) Anorectal anomalies. In: Spitz L, Coran AG, eds. _Paediatric Surgery_. 5th edn. Chapman and Hall, London: 423–51

Pokorny WJ (1995) Necrotising enterocolitis. In: Spitz L, Coran AG, eds. _Paediatric Surgery_. 5th edn. Chapman and Hall, London: 411–23

Roback S (1988) Common conditions requiring gastrointestinal stomas in infants. _J Enterostomal Ther_ 15: 162–6

Rogers VE(2003) Managing preemie stomas, more than just a pouch. _J Wound Care Nurs_ 30(2): 100–11

Webster P (1985) Special babies. _Community Outlook_ 5: 20–2

Williams C (1999) _An investigation of the benefits of Aquacel Hydrofiber® wound dressing. Br J Nurs_ 8(10): 676–80

Williams J, Nichols RJ (undated) _Ulcerative colitis, a surgical guide for parents._ St Marks Hospital Information Booklet, London

Lyon CC, Beck M (2001) Irritant reactions and allergy. Chap 3: 41–96. In: Lyon CC, Smith AJ, eds. _Abdominal Stomas and their Skin Disorders. An atlas of diagnosis and management._ Martin Dunitz, London

Recommended reading

Black PK (2000) *Holistic Stoma Care*. Baillière Tindall, Edinburgh, London: chap 18

Lyon CC, Smith AJ, eds. *Abdominal Stomas and their Skin Disorders. An atlas of diagnosis and management*. Martin Dunitz, London

Chapter 10

Epidermolysis bullosa

Jacqueline Denyer

Epidermolysis bullosa (EB) is the term given to a large group of genetically determined skin disorders in which the common factor is fragility of the skin and mucous membranes (Lin and Carter, 1992).

There is a wide range of severity, varying between mild discomfort and death in early infancy.

Management of children and adults with epidermolysis bullosa is complex and for those severely affected requires a multidisciplinary approach to care in a specialised centre. In addition to the main team, all personnel in contact with the child must be trained in specific handling techniques.

General guidelines for management of the child with severe epidermolysis bullosa

The principles of care are:

❖ Employ specialised handling techniques to reduce the risks of increased skin blistering and wounds resulting from friction and shearing forces.
❖ Remove labels from clothing. Choose flat-seamed under garments, or turn clothing inside out to ensure prominent seams do not rub and cause blisters.

❖ Avoid use of adhesive tapes. Mepitac® (Mölnlycke Health Care) is a safe alternative and suitable for securing intravenous cannulae, nasogastric tubes and dressings. Where adhesive tape has been applied by accident, or it is essential to use adhesive products for accurate monitoring of vital signs, safe removal can be achieved without skin damage by using 50% liquid/50% white soft paraffin, or a non-sting commercial medical adhesive remover such as Appeel® (Clinimed).

Care of the neonate

The following factors need to be considered and addressed when caring for neonates.

❖ Neonates are especially vulnerable and transferring them to a specialised centre may involve travelling a long distance, resulting in a great deal of unnecessary skin loss. To avoid this, specialised nurses will take diagnostic samples and teach handling, feeding and dressing techniques to staff and parents in the referring unit. Community nurses are trained prior to the infant's discharge home (Denyer, 2000).
❖ The infant can be reviewed at a specialised centre once the inter-utero and birth damage have healed.
❖ Heat and humidity encourage blistering, therefore neonates and infants should be nursed in an open cot or bassinette, unless incubator care is required for medical reasons such as prematurity.
❖ Remove the cord clamp and replace with a ligature to protect the peri-umbilical skin from erosions.
❖ It is essential that all routine screening for congenital abnormalities is carried out, but techniques will need modification to reduce skin loss and blistering. Blood sampling via a heel prick should be avoided and venopuncture technique employed. Unless there are concerns for the infant's longer term survival, samples for DNA analysis should be deferred until the time of the Guthrie test to avoid additional venopuncture. Congenital dislocation of the hips should be excluded using ultrasound imagery rather than manipulation.

❖ Identification bands should not be placed around limbs as these can rub, bands should be attached to clothing.

❖ Blisters must be lanced with a hypodermic needle; blisters on the skin of those with EB are not self-limiting and will continue to enlarge if not ruptured (*Figure 10.1*). The roof should be left on the blister. Apply cornflour to help dry the blister and reduce friction. Cornflour is chemically inert and water soluble and will not cause irritation if it comes in contact with mucous membranes. This practice has been used extensively in the author's unit for ten years with no reported ill effects.

❖ When caring for children with a genetic skin disorder, be aware that many dressings described as 'non-adherent' by the manufacturer may behave differently on the skin of those affected.

❖ Pain management should follow individual assessment using a recognised tool.

❖ Increased nutrients are required where there is a large amount of skin loss. Specialised teats may be required as a sore mouth will make the infant reluctant to feed (*Figure 10.2*).

❖ Gastro-oesophageal reflux is a feature in all types of EB. The acid from stomach contents can increase mouth and oesophageal blistering, increasing the risk of oesophageal strictures in severe cases.

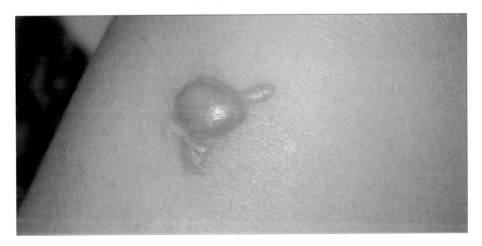

Figure 10.1: Blisters will spread if not lanced

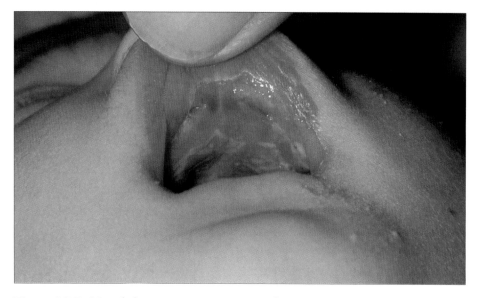

Figure 10.2: Mouth lesions in a neonate with severe EB

Types of epidermolysis bullosa

There are three main groups of epidermolysis bullosa:

- epidermolysis simplex (EBS)
- junctional epidermolysis bullosa (JEB)
- dystrophic epidermolysis bullosa (DEB).

Within each group there are many subtypes, each with a varying prognosis.

Other genodermatoses, including bullous ichthyosiform erythroderma and Kindler disease, share the characteristics of skin fragility and blistering, but are not strictly classified as types of EB and their management will not be discussed for the purpose of this chapter.

Initial diagnosis is made from analysis of a shave skin biopsy taken from gently rubbed clinically unaffected skin. Interpretation of the biopsy should be carried out at a diagnostic centre with a specific remit for epidermolysis bullosa. The type of EB is determined by the level of split within the skin seen on electron microscopy. Further categorisation can often be achieved following molecular studies.

Epidermolysis bullosa simplex (EBS)

Epidermolysis bullosa simplex is generally a dominantly inherited condition, often with extensive family history. One parent will be affected and there is a 1:2 risk in every pregnancy that the baby will be similarly affected. _De novo_ mutations occur when neither parent is affected but a mutation occurs in a single egg or sperm.

There are 3 main types of EB simplex:

- Weber-Cockayne
- Köebner
- Dowling Meara.

All of these are dominantly inherited and have defects in the proteins keratin 5 or 14.

Rarer types of EBS are recessively inherited, both parents will be unaffected carriers and there is a 1:4 risk in every pregnancy that the baby will be affected. The most severe form of recessive simplex is EBS with muscular dystrophy; the defect is located in the plectin protein which is also expressed in muscular tissue.

EBS Weber-Cockayne primarily affects the hands and feet with blisters arising readily in response to humid conditions. Where some individuals are affected all year round, others blister only in the summer months. The prevalence is estimated at 5–20 affected individuals per million.

Management is by lancing the blisters and use of dressings with a cooling effect, such as hydrogels. Shoes are not well tolerated and should be made from soft leather with no internal seams, children require several pairs of shoes to be worn in rotation to alter the sites of blistering. Vulnerable areas of skin can be protected by silicone dressings. Socks containing a silver thread are commercially available and help reduce heat. Socks and shoes can be stored in plastic bags in the refrigerator to help cool the feet and reduce the rate of blistering. Mobility may be severely compromised due to pain, and many children need a wheelchair for several days each week to allow healing of blistered areas before they are able to walk again.

The Köebner-type of EBS has a pattern of more widespread blistering and skin fragility. Management is similar to those with the Weber-Cockayne type. Prevalence of the Köebner EBS is estimated at two per million.

EBS Dowling Meara is frequently seen as a *de novo* mutation in the absence of family history. Prevalence is estimated at 5–10 per million. This type of EB can have serious implications and there is a significant mortality rate in the neonatal period, arising from complications such as sepsis. Longer term problems include severe gastro-oesophageal reflux with feeding difficulties and hoarseness of voice due to laryngeal blistering. In general, the extensive blistering reduces over time, although a later problem is the development of hyperkeratosis over the palms and soles and thickened nails (*Figure 10.3*). In a few individuals there is marked disability persisting into adulthood (McGrath *et al*, 1992).

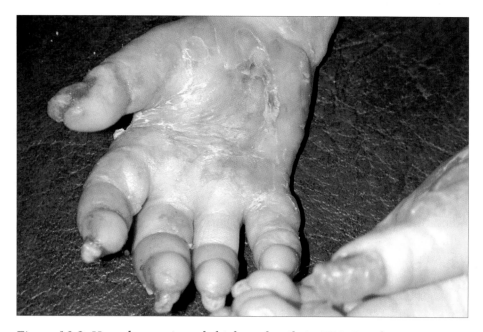

Figure 10.3: Hyperkeratosis and thickened nails in EBS, Dowling Meara

Unlike other types of EB, children with Dowling Meara are frequently unable to tolerate dressings as these exacerbate blistering, particularly around the edges of the dressing. Where there is an open wound, dressings should be light and soft such as Hydrofiber® dressings (ConvaTec), held in place with a tubular retention bandage. Dressings should be withheld as soon as possible and, while in place, removed frequently to lance fresh blisters which form beneath them.

EBS with associated muscular dystrophy results from a defect of plectin protein. The prevalence is uncertain, but this is an extremely rare type of EB. Skin involvement may be minimal but laryngeal blistering and subsequent scarring may require insertion of tracheostomy. Muscle weakness is progressive leading to wheelchair dependency and reduced life expectancy (Mellerio _et al_, 1997).

Junctional epidermolysis bullosa (JEB)

Junctional EB has 3 main subtypes:

- Herlitz
- non-Herlitz
- JEB with pyloric atresia.

All forms of junctional EB are recessively inherited. Prevalence is difficult to interpret because of the high early mortality rate often before diagnosis can be made. Within the UK, incidence is estimated at 20 per million births.

Herlitz junctional epidermolysis bullosa (HJEB) results from a defect in the protein laminin 5 and is usually the most serious type of EB, with few infants surviving beyond the first year life, and the majority dying within their first few weeks or months. Death results from a combination of laryngeal disease and failure to thrive, frequently in combination with sepsis. Rapid blistering develops following gentle handling and large areas of ulceration soon appear. Finger and toe nails are lost within the first few days or weeks of life, leaving open nail beds which require careful dressing (_Figure 10.4_).

Extensive dressings may be required by those severely affected. Soft silicone products in the main are well tolerated and are non-adherent. (Williams, 1995; White, 2005).

Healing is slow and will not be achieved in those who fail to thrive.

Short-term potent topical steroid treatment can be very successful in healing over-granulating wounds.

Non-Herlitz JEB results from a defect in laminin 5 or type XV11 collagen. This type of EB varies in its severity. Some children have few areas of ulceration, while others have large open wounds typically located on the lower legs and scalp. Hair loss is common in those with non-Herlitz JEB.

JEB with an associated pyloric atresia results from a protein defect within integrin $\alpha 6$ $\beta 4$ and carries an extremely poor prognosis, with the majority of infants not surviving beyond the neonatal period. Surgical correction of the atresia is generally successful, but there are sometimes associated renal abnormalities. There are, however, a few longer term survivors who have nail dystrophy but few other skin problems.

All the longer term survivors with JEB are at risk of blistering within the mucosa of the bladder and urethra, leading to stricture formation, dysuria and eventually retention. Affected children may require supra pubic urinary drainage or, in extreme cases, diversionary surgery in the form of a mitroffanof.

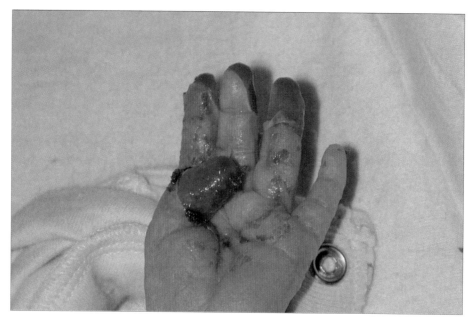

Figure 10.4: Typical lesions on the fingers of a neonate with Herlitz JEB

Dystrophic epidermolysis bullosa (DEB)

Dystrophic epidermolysis bullosa results from a defect in collagen 7. The skin is deficient in anchoring fibrils and any shearing force causes the skin to strip away.

DEB may be dominant or recessively inherited. Prevalence in the UK is unclear, an estimated prevalence in Scotland was 21.4 per million for all types of DEB. Carrier frequency for recessive dystrophic EB is thought to be 1:350 (Murata-Takayuki *et al*, 2004).

In common with many other genetically determined conditions, those with the dominant form tend to be more mildly affected. However, there is a large scale of severity in those with the recessive type.

Severely affected infants are often born with large areas of denuded skin typically over the feet and lower legs, resulting from trauma of the infant kicking *in utero*. These wounds can show both previous signs of healing and fresh trauma. Damage is compounded by the trauma of delivery. Those born via caesarean section may have less extensive damage at birth, but this does not necessarily indicate a milder form of the disease.

Dressings may be required to cover most of the body and a full dressing change can take several hours. Dressings are selected which will not require changing daily or where at least the primary dressing can be left in place. Exudate and odour management are frequently required.

Soft silicone products are well tolerated (*Figure 10.5*) and can also be used as a non-adherent wound contact layer in order to use therapeutic dressings.

Lipidohydrocolloid dressings covered with foam dressings are useful when intact vulnerable skin requires protection from trauma (Blanchet-Bardon and Bohot, 2005).

Exudate poses a particular problem as the peri-wound skin is extraordinarily fragile. Capillary action dressings and highly absorptive dressings can be used successfully, but must be placed on top of a soft silicone dressing to ensure non-adherence. Such dressings can also cause skin tearing due to the weight of the dressing pulling on the skin on a vertical surface such as the child's back.

Odour is a common feature and can result in children being ostracised at school. Charcoal dressings are effective to an extent, but better control has been achieved recently using honey. Honey has also demonstrated an ability to heal chronic wounds in those with EB, but the initial increase in exudate has proved intolerable for some children (Hon, 2005).

Wound infections are common and systemic infections such as streptococci require antibiotic therapy. Topical antibiotics are discouraged because of the high incidence of resistant organisms (Moy *et al*, 1990). A prolonged course of oral antibiotics is often necessary to ensure effective treatment.

Critical colonisation delays wound healing but generally responds to topical antimicrobials (Cutting, 2003), of which we find silver sulfadiazine and 1% stabilised hydrogen peroxide being used in rotation to be well tolerated with minimal risk of resistance.

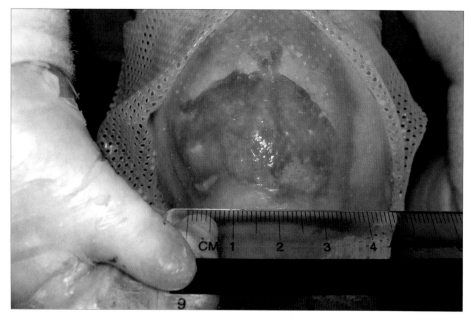

Figure 10.5: Atraumatic removal of Mepitel® (Mölnlycke Health Care) soft silicone dressing in recessive dystrophic EB

Many children experience intractable pruritis which causes extreme discomfort and damage to the skin. Children are frequently seen with an intact area of the skin in the centre of their back, which has been spared excoriation and skin loss because the child cannot reach to scratch.

Antihistamines appear to have little effect. Measures such as creating a cool environment and wearing cotton clothing help to a limited extent. Weak topical steroid application has proved helpful and can be used in combination with a wet wrap technique, provided open wounds are first protected with a non-adherent dressing to prevent adhesion to the tubular bandage.

Over time, the lesions heal with a contractural scar leading to reduced mobility. Regular physiotherapy can help to maintain mobility but wheelchair dependency is not uncommon in older children. Electric wheelchairs provide pain-free mobility and are popular when children wish to keep up with their peers. However, our experience shows children's ability to mobilise independently rapidly reduces after the introduction of electric wheelchairs and we recommend these for limited use only.

Finger and toe nails may be absent at birth or be gradually lost over the first few weeks or months, the bed is healed beneath the nail bed and poses little problems apart from reduced fine motor skills, such as opening packaging. Hand function is progressively reduced in those severely affected as continual blistering and trauma lead to scarring and contractures. Digital fusion develops as the web spaces are gradually lost (Fine *et al*, 2005b).

'Degloving' injuries follow gentle restraint for procedures such as venepuncture in the neonate (*Figure 10.6*), a fall on an outstretched hand or when a child trips when holding the hand of another child or adult. Degloving injuries require careful dressing and splinting to avoid rapid progression to contractures and fusion of the fingers. Formation of contractures can be delayed by regular exercising and splinting. Unfortunately, splints are not always well tolerated as the children use them to scratch with and cause extensive damage to the skin and sometimes rub their eyes leading to corneal abrasions. Surgery to separate the fingers and release the contractures can be successfully done, but will need to be repeated when hand function again deteriorates. Older children and adults frequently refuse this surgery as the benefits are short-lived, provided the first web space remains, opposed function is surprisingly good (*Figure 10.7*).

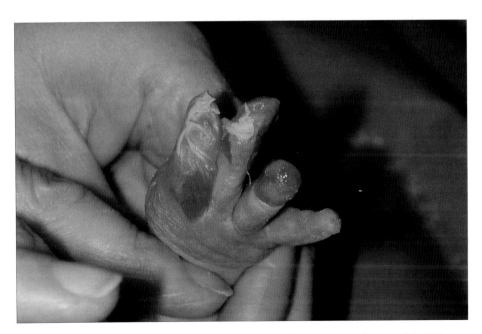

Figure 10.6: Degloving injuries in neonate with recessive dystrophic EB

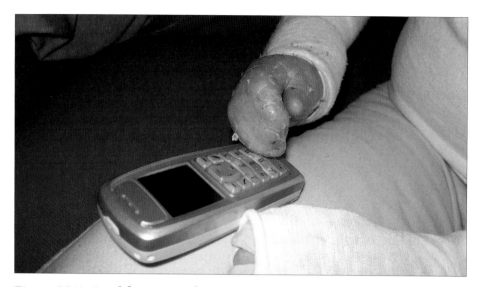

Figure 10.7: Good fine motor function despite digital fusion and contractures in severe recessive dystrophic EB

Prognosis varies in those with the severe form of dystrophic EB. The majority survive into early- or mid-adulthood but with increasing disability. Death usually results from squamous cell carcinoma. These are multiple primaries with rapid progression towards secondary tumours. Management is by surgical excision; radiotherapy and chemotherapy are not very effective but may be used in palliative treatment. Survival rate following the first tumour is on average only 5 years (Yamada *et al*, 2004).

Common problems in severe EB

Dental

Dental decay is a common factor in children with severe EB. Those with the junctional type have enamel hypoplasia leading to rapid decay, and reconstruction is necessary for the longer term survivors (Kirkham *et al*, 2000).

While children with dystrophic EB have normal tooth structure, microstomia leads to overcrowding and this, together with a reluctance to brush teeth effectively due to fragile mucosa, leads to decay (Harris _et al_, 2001).

Nutrition

Children with severe EB require additional nutrients to compensate for blood and plasma loss from wounds, frequent skin infections and continual wound healing. Unfortunately, in those with the dystrophic form of EB, intake is restricted from a combination of mechanical difficulties caused by microstomia, tethering of the tongue from scar tissue, dental overcrowding, and decay and dysphagia resulting from oesophageal strictures. Repeated dilatations reduce dysphagia but, in addition to these, some children require supplementary gastrostomy feeding (Haynes _et al_, 1996; Anderson _et al_, 2004).

Appetite is further reduced by chronic constipation, resulting from reluctance to pass stools due to pain from peri-anal blistering and fissures. Osmotic laxatives containing polyethylene glycol have proved effective in managing constipation. Enemas and suppositories should be avoided because of the risk of trauma exacerbating the problem.

Severe anaemia results from constant blood loss both from wounds and mucous membranes. In addition to oral iron supplements, children may require blood transfusions or intravenous iron infusions. Venous access is poor due to scarring and contractures, but in-dwelling aids such as ports and lines have proved difficult to keep free from infection.

Dilated cardiomyopathy is a rare complication in children with severe EB (Melville _et al_, 1996). This may prove to be fatal, but there are a small number of children who have improved following supplementation with selenium, suggesting that compromised nutrition may predispose this condition (Sidwell _et al_, 2000).

Pain management

Pain management is difficult in epidermolysis bullosa due to the variation in symptoms on any one day, and the multiple contributing factors (Weiner, 2004).

Pain is assessed using a recognised tool which includes behavioural and cultural characteristics (Herod _et al_, 2002). Mild pain generally responds to simple analgesia such as paracetamol, combined with a non-steroidal. Severe pain requires treatment with an opioid analgesia which can be combined with an anxiolytic such as midazolam. Chronic background pain must be considered and can be managed by introduction of a long-acting opioid. Topical opioids are effective in the management of wounds in some children (Watterson *et al*, 2004).

Even in those with a mild form of EB, there is an element of neuropathic pain which is managed by low dose amitriptylline or gabapentin.

Eyes

Corneal ulceration develops following blistering and erosions (Fine *et al*, 2004). This is very painful and the child is extremely photosensitive requiring regular analgesia and to stay in a darkened room until the lesion has healed. Conjunctival scarring may follow repeated injuries and can reduce vision. Artificial tears must be given regularly to maintain the tear film, particularly for those with the dystrophic form, where scarring of the eyelids prohibits complete closure of the eye.

Psychosocial effects

In its severe forms EB is a painful, disfiguring and progressive disabling condition. Affected children and their families require ongoing psychological support to help develop coping strategies. There is a high rate of divorce and separation among parents of severely affected children (Fine *et al*, 2005a).

Some severely affected adults have developed lifestyles and care packages which allow for successful independent living (Hall, 2004).

Those less severely affected feel that they have a hidden disability and may not receive the necessary support they require.

The future

The molecular pathology for all types of EB has been identified and work is progressing towards gene therapy (Ferrari *et al*, 2005). *Ex vivo* techniques using gene corrected keratinocytes grafted onto wound sites have been successfully carried out on animal models in the laboratory. However, this method does not offer hope for correcting gastrointestinal complications.

Pre-natal diagnosis is now available for those at risk of having children with a severe form of junctional or dystrophic EB. In the majority of cases this follows analysis of extracted DNA from a chorionic villous sample taken in early pregnancy (McGrath *et al*, 1996). Occasionally, genetic mutations cannot be identified and diagnosis is made by analysis of a fetal skin biopsy taken in the second trimester.

Techniques are now available to offer pre-gestational diagnosis using *in vitro* fertilisation with DNA analysis from one cell of the 8 cell balstomere.

Case study 1

Lucy was born via normal vaginal delivery at 39 weeks gestation, following an uneventful pregnancy. She is the second child of unrelated parents. Her parents were horrified to see that there was no skin on her feet and lower legs. In the minutes following her birth, blisters appeared on her face when the midwife dried her with a soft towel and oral suction caused blood to ooze from her mouth.

Staff in the maternity unit were very distressed. It was thought Lucy had contracted an inter-uterine infection and a cannula was sited in the back of her hand for administration of intravenous antibiotics. Her legs were gently wrapped in Vaseline gauze and she was placed in an incubator in the special care baby unit for observation.

Over the next few days her condition worsened. She was nursed naked and removed skin over her chest as a result of rubbing her arms against it. Feeding caused her sore mouth to blister badly and a nasogastric tube was inserted to maintain her nutrition.

The cannula needed to be replaced but when the securing tape was removed the skin on her hand stripped away leaving an open wound. She cried constantly despite receiving regular opioid analgesia.

A differential diagnosis of epidermolysis bullosa was made and a referral made to a specialist centre. A specialist nurse visited Lucy the following day and made a clinic diagnosis of epidermolysis bullosa (EB). A diagnostic skin biopsy was taken and her wounds were dressed with appropriate non-adherent dressings. The cannula and nasogastric tube were not required and the adhesive tape removed without skin stripping by using medical adhesive remover. Parents and staff were shown how to handle and feed Lucy without risk of additional skin trauma.

Her parents were informed of the diagnosis and given an explanation of the three main types of EB. Written information was left for them.

Analysis of the skin biopsy determined that Lucy has recessive dystrophic EB. She will develop multiple problems resulting from scarring of her skin, eyes and mucous membranes. Her mobility will be reduced as contractures increase and fine motor skills hampered by increasing pseudo-syndactyly.

She will require support from her specialist EB nurses, community team, local hospital and the multidisciplinary team at her specialist hospital.

Her parents received genetic counselling and will be offered pre-natal testing in any future pregnancies.

Case study 2

Liz has EB simplex (EBS), Weber Cockayne type. Her hands and feet blister in the summer months, and this limits her mobility as the blisters are very painful. She has learnt to restrict her lifestyle so she walks as little as possible. She drives to work and sits at her desk for most of the day, taking her shoes off under the desk as they put pressure on the blisters and make her feet sore.

Her first child, Luke, was born in November. There is a strong family history of EBS and Liz knew that there was a one in two risk that the baby would inherit EB. She had received genetic counselling and knew the type of EB would be the same as her own and not one of the more serious types.

When Luke was born, Liz examined him for signs of blistering. She even rubbed his skin to see if she could induce blistering.

There were no signs that Luke had inherited EB and Liz was cautiously optimistic.

Luke started walking at 13 months of age and still his feet did not blister. Liz now felt he definitely did not have EB.

The following summer, when Luke was 19 months old he was playing in the garden on a hot day when he started to cry. Liz took off his shoes and, to her horror, found that his feet were covered in blisters. She took him to her GP and Luke was referred to a specialised centre for EB. While she waited for an appointment, Liz managed Luke's blisters in same way as her own — lancing them with a sewing needle which she had sterilised by boiling it on the hob and applying antiseptic cream and wrapping his feet in open weave bandages. The bandages were soaked off in the bath every night.

When Luke was seen in the specialised centre, Liz was amazed at the progress in dressings which had been made since she was a child. They were prescribed hypodermic needles to lance the blisters, and soothing non-adherent dressings. Liz was advised to give pain relief regularly when his feet were blistered. The podiatrist offered advice on suitable footwear.

Luke will have an annual appointment in which they will be shown any available new products and his pain management will be assessed.

Liz was referred to a specialised centre for adults to update her own care.

References

Anderson S, Meenan J, Williams K *et al* (2004) Efficacy and safety of endoscopic dilatation of oesophageal strictures in epidermolysis bullosa. *Gastrointestinal Endoscopy* **59**(1): 28–32

Blanchet-Bardon C, Bohot S (2005) Using Urgotul dressing for the management of epidermolysis bullosa skin lesions. *J Wound Care* **14**(10): 490–1, 494–6

Cutting KF (2003) Wound healing, bacteria and topical therapies. *EWMA J* **3**(1): 17–19

Denyer J (2000) Management of severe blistering disorders. *Semin Neonatol* **5**(4): 321–4

Ferrari S, Pellegrini G, Mavilio F, Deluca M (2005) Gene therapy approaches for epidermolysis bullosa. *Clin Dermatol* **23**(4): 430–6

Fine JD, Johnson L, Weiner M (2004) Eye involvement in inherited epidermolysis bullosa: experience of the National Epidermolysis Bullosa Registry. *Am J Ophthalmol* **138**(2): 254–62

Fine JD, Johnson LB, Weiner M (2005a) Impact of inherited epidermolysis bullosa on parental interpersonal relationships, marital status and family size. *Br J Dermatol* **152**(5): 1009–14

Fine JD, Johnson LB, Weiner M *et al* (2005b) Pseudosyndactyly and musculoskeletal contractures in inherited epidermolysis bullosa: experience of the National Epidermolysis Bullosa Registry, 1986–2002. *J Hand Surg* **30**(1): 14–22

Hall S (2004) Life, epidermolysis bullosa and chasing tornadoes. *J Wound Care* **13**(10): 405–6

Harris JC, Bryan RA, Lucas VS, Roberts GJ (2001) Dental disease and caries related micro flora in children with dystrophic epidermolysis bullosa. *Pediatr Dentistry* **23**(5): 438–43

Haynes L, Atherton DJ, Ade-Ajaye N *et al* (1996) Gastrostomy and growth in dystrophic epidermolysis bullosa. *Br J Dermatol* **134**(5): 872–9

Herod J, Denyer J, Goldman A, Howard R (2002) Epidermolysis bullosa in children, pathophysiology, anaesthesia and pain management. *Paediatr Anaesth* **11**(5): 388–97

Hon J (2005) Using honey to heal a chronic wound in a patient with epidermolysis bullosa. *Br J Nurs* **14**(19) Tissue viability supplement: S4–S12

Kirkham J, Robinson C, Strafford SM *et al* (2000) The chemical composition of tooth enamel in junctional epidermolysis bullosa. *Arch Oral Biology* **45**(5): 377–86

Lin AN, Carter DM (1992) *Epidermolysis Bullosa: Basic and Clinical Aspects.* Springer Verlag, New York

McGrath JA, Ishida-Yamamoo, Tidman MJ *et al* (1992) Epidermolysis bullosa simplex (Dowling Meara): a clinicopathological review. *Br J Dermatol* **126**: 421–30

McGrath JA, Dunnill MG, Christiano AM *et al* (1996) First trimester DNA-based exclusion of recessive dystrophic epidermolysis bullosa from chorionic villus sampling. *Br J Dermatol* **134**(4): 734–9

Mellerio JE, Smith FJD, McMillan JR *et al* (1997) Recessive epidermolysis bullosa simplex associated with plectin mutations: infantile respiratory complications in two unrelated cases. *Br J Dermatol* **137**: 898–906

Melville C, Atherton D, Burch M *et al* (1996) Fatal cardiomyopathy in dystrophic epidermolysis bullosa. *Br J Dermatol* **135**(4): 603–6

Moy JA, Caldwell-Brown D, Lina AN *et al* (1990) Mupirocin-resistant *Staphylococcus aureus* after long-term treatment of patients with epidermolysis bullosa. *J Am Dermatol* **22**: 893–5

Murata-Takayuki, Masunager-Takuji, Ishiko-Akira *et al* (2004) Differences in recurrent COL7A1 mutations in dystrophic epidermolysis bullosa ethnic-specific and worldwide recurrent mutations. *Arch Dermatological Res* **295**(10): 442–7

Sidwell R, Yates R, Atherton DJ (2000) Dilated cardiomyopathy in dystrophic epidermolysis bullosa. *Arch Dis Childhood* **83**(1): 59–63

Watterson G, Howard R, Goldman A (2004) Peripheral options in inflammatory pain. *Arch Dis Childhood* **89**(7): 679–81

Weiner M (2004) Pain management in epidermolysis bullosa: an intractable problem. *Ostomy/Wound Management* **50**(8): 13–14

White R (2005) Evidence for atraumatic soft silicone wound dressing use. *Wounds UK* **1**(3): 104–9

Williams C (1995) Mepitel. *Br J Nurs* **4**(1): 51–2, 54–5

Yamada-Mizuki, Hatta-Naohito, Sogo-Kana *et al* (2004) Management of squamous cell carcinoma in a patient with recessive type epidermolysis bullosa dystrophica. *Dermatological Surg* **30**(11): 1424–9

Chapter 11

Preventing trauma and pain in paediatric wound care

Fiona Burton, Valerie Irving and Elaine Bethell

Preventing trauma and pain in paediatric wound care is a challenge for many different healthcare professionals and this has been amplified in recent years due to the increased rate of survival of premature neonates. Infants who are born prematurely are at increased risk of developing skin trauma and associated complications (McManus Kuller *et al*, 2002). Furthermore, evidence suggests that neonates are more sensitive to pain than older children and adults (Anand, 1998; Johnston *et al*, 1999; Anand *et al*, 2001), and this can cause long-term developmental or behavioural effects (Porter *et al*, 1999). However, management of pain is hindered by the lack of awareness among some healthcare professionals that neonates actually feel pain (de Lima *et al*, 1996), and anxiety among carers concerning the possible adverse effects of analgesia (Anand *et al*, 2001). This is further exacerbated by the limited evidence base behind paediatric wound care practice and pain management, because of the ethical issues involved in carrying out clinical studies on this population.

This chapter provides an overview of the risk factors associated with neonatal skin, the causes of trauma and pain in paediatric wound care, the assessment of pain, and the prevention or management of trauma and pain.

Increased risk factors for neonatal skin

Although epidermal development is complete by the end of the second trimester of pregnancy (20–24 weeks), there is little or no water permeability barrier function at this time (Hardman *et al*, 1999) (see *Chapter 1, Figure 1.3, p. 7*). Consequently, the barrier function of the skin in premature infants is minimal and the neonates are exposed to a number of risk factors (McManus Kuller *et al*, 2002). These include high transepidermal water loss, which can be as much as 15 times greater in pre-term children compared with full-term, leading to excessive heat loss from the constantly damp skin (Rutter, 1996). Furthermore, the compromised barrier means that there is increased potential for chemicals to be absorbed through the skin and the infants are more susceptible to infection (Rutter, 1996).

Neonates are also vulnerable to iatrogenic tissue damage (Rutter, 2000; Irving, 2001a) caused by monitoring probes and care procedures. The dermis does not fully develop until after birth and, even at full-term, it is only 60% of its adult thickness (Wysocki, 2000). The fibrils connecting the epidermis and dermis are reduced in number and are more widely spaced in neonatal skin, leaving it vulnerable to shear forces, and it is easily damaged or removed, especially by adhesive products (epidermal stripping) (Irving, 2001a).

At 24 weeks gestation, the skin appears moist, shiny and red because of the lack of subcutaneous fat between the dermis and muscle tissue (Irving, 2001a). Subcutaneous fat does not begin to develop until 29 weeks gestation. However, exposure to air accelerates maturation of the neonatal skin so that, no matter how premature the infant, within two weeks the skin will have developed to the same extent as that of a full-term infant (Evans and Rutter, 1986).

Preventing trauma and pain

Pain has been defined as 'an unpleasant sensory and emotional experience associated with actual or potential tissue damage, or described in terms of such damage' (Merskey and Bogduk, 1994). The most obvious and effective method to reduce pain associated with wounds is to prevent the wound occurring in the first place. The immaturity of neonatal skin means that premature infants are particularly susceptible to a number of specific types of wounds, and many of these are preventable if simple measures are implemented (Association of Women's Health, Obstetric and Neonatal Nurses [AWHONN], 2001; Irving, 2001a). The practitioner should assess each child's risk of developing tissue damage and implement preventative care; the goal being to maintain skin integrity (McManus Kuller, 2001).

Managing specific wounds in neonates and paediatrics

Epidermal stripping

Epidermal stripping is a particular risk for neonates born before 27 weeks gestation (Irving, 2001a). Skin damage can easily occur, for example, when removing adhesive tapes that are used to secure tubes or dressings, as these products may bond to the epidermis more strongly than the epidermis does with the dermis (Gunderson and Kenner, 1995). All tape should be evaluated before use and the minimum amount necessary applied (Malloy-McDonald, 1995).

Clear film dressings should be used to secure intravenous (IV) cannulae, as they allow monitoring of the site without removal. An alcohol-free skin barrier film applied beneath the film dressing may also help to reduce skin stripping (Irving, 2001b). In some cases, handling alone may cause epidermal stripping, and it is important to ensure that nails are kept short and all stoned rings are taken off, as these can cause damage to the vulnerable skin. Splints used to support IV cannulae can be secured using Velcro® strapping as an alternative to adhesive tapes, but the site must always be visible.

Chemical burns

Chemical burns can be caused by contact between alcohol-based skin preparation solutions and neonatal skin (Harpin and Rutter,

1982; Watkins and Keogh, 1992). If these agents are applied before insertion of umbilical lines, IV cannulae or drains, they should be rinsed off immediately with sterile water. However, it is better to avoid them totally and instead use aqueous-based skin preparations such as chlorhexidine (West *et al*, 1981). All solutions should be applied sparingly and exposure limited, as over-generous application can result in the baby lying on alcohol-saturated bedding during the procedure, which can lead to full-thickness burns due to the prolonged contact. Repeated use of iodine-based solutions can cause hypothyroidism due to iodine absorption and should be avoided in the pre-term infant (Linder *et al*, 1997).

Thermal injuries

Thermal injuries can be caused by heat from monitoring electrodes or, more rarely, the fibre optic 'cold light' used to identify veins or arteries for insertion of cannulae or central lines. Burns from electrodes that heat the skin (to cause dilation of blood vessels for monitoring of transcutaneous O_2 and CO_2), can be avoided by reducing the temperature and the length of their application time, according to the age and gestation of the neonate (Gunderson and Kenner, 1995). Cold light burns may be prevented by minimising usage time of the fibre optic light, and using a protective guard will prevent direct contact with the skin.

Pressure/ischaemic injuries

Pressure/ischaemic injuries occasionally occur in neonates and older children. Infants who are sedated or paralysed and, therefore, unable to make spontaneous movements are at risk of pressure injuries (Gunderson and Kenner, 1995). Children with low blood pressure and receiving inotropes are also at increased risk, as this medication causes vasoconstriction in peripheral blood vessels in an effort to improve the blood pressure. The reduction in blood flow to the peripheries can result in poor perfusion, increasing the risk of pressure damage (Lund, 1999). This can also occur with oedematous babies.

Pressure ulcers or ischaemic injuries may occur on the ears or the occiput, if the child is nursed supine, or on the knees, if nursed prone. A programme for repositioning babies should be developed to prevent pressure ulcers or ischaemic injuries occurring. Pressure-reducing surfaces that are suitable for incubators and cots will reduce the risk further. These include gel/viscous fluid pads, air-filled mattresses and pressure-redistributing foam mattresses (Lund, 1999). Pressure ulcers may also be avoided by making sure that infants are not lying on tubing, and by using IV cannulae that do not have wings. Saturation probes should be repositioned every 3–4 hours or, more frequently, for very pre-term babies (National Association for Neonatal Nurses [NANN], 1997).

If the baby is receiving nasal continuous positive airway pressure (CPAP), care must be taken to ensure that the nasal prongs fit correctly and that the pressure under the prongs is relieved on a regular basis, otherwise damage may occur to the nasal septum (Glynn, 2004). There are no set recommendations for the frequency with which this must be done, so it should be performed on an individual basis. Babies may become oedematous post-delivery and, if this occurs, clothing or tapes must be loosened to reduce the risk of pressure ulcers developing.

Extravasation injuries

Extravasation injuries occur when vesicant fluid inadvertently leaks from a vein/cannula site into surrounding tissue. This leakage can be caused by dislodgement of the tip of the cannula, or puncturing of the vein, and quick action is essential to minimise further injury. Children most at risk of extravasation injury include those receiving IV caffeine, glucose (>10%), calcium, or total parenteral nutrition (TPN), particularly when this is given through a peripheral line (Blatz and Paes, 1990). Infants receiving hypertonic solutions (Hecker, 1993) or IV inotropes, which cause vasoconstriction, are also at risk.

Ensuring that the cannula is carefully sited, using tributaries of the cephalic and basilic veins on the dorsum of the hand, the dorsal venous arch, and the medial and lateral marginal veins in the foot, can reduce the risk of these injuries occurring. Scalp veins should be used only as a last resort as shaving off the hair around the area is necessary and cannulae are difficult to secure (Blatz and Paes, 1990).

Sterile transparent film dressings should be used to secure the line, thus allowing good observation of the site. Although the median life span of an IV cannula in neonates is 36 hours (Hecker *et al*, 1991), the tip may become obstructed by fibrin or thrombin, especially if left in place for too long. Therefore, lines should be checked for signs of leakage, dislodgement, swelling, oedema or blanching, at least hourly, so that the practitioner is able to respond quickly to any reduction in patency (Bravery, 1999).

Ischaemic injuries

As stated above, ischaemic injuries can result from extravasation of a peripheral arterial line but, more frequently, they will be caused by arterial spasm. Inspection of arterial lines every 30–60 minutes is recommended and, once a problem has been identified, the line should be removed immediately. A loss of trace on the blood pressure transducers that are attached to peripheral arterial lines indicates that the line is not functioning properly, and any difficulty in sampling blood from the line may suggest a predisposition to arterial spasm, or clot formation, and the line should be removed to prevent an ischaemic injury from occurring.

During the antenatal period, amniotic banding injuries can occur. This rare birth condition is caused by rupture of the amniotic sac early in the pregnancy, which leaves the developing fetus exposed to the placenta's fibrous tissues. These can become entangled with the developing limbs, acting as a tourniquet as the baby grows and causing varying degrees of damage that, ultimately, may result in poorly perfused or ischaemic and gangrenous limbs. Immediate surgery may be required in these cases to save the affected limb or digit.

Surgical wounds

Surgical wounds in paediatrics are often closed subcutaneously (with no external sutures), or sutured and covered with a film dressing so that the wound site is visible. It is important that these wounds are viewed with each set of care procedures for signs of infection (such as redness, swelling, increased exudate, or the presence of pus) that can prevent the wound from healing, and all assessments documented appropriately.

Pain is a classic symptom of wound infection, but, because young infants cannot vocalise their pain, staff must observe for signs of extreme quietness; facial actions, such as brow bulge or eyes squeezed shut; a change in heart or respiratory rate; increased oxygen requirements; or intolerance of feeds (American Academy of Pediatrics/Canadian Paediatric Society, 2000).

Film dressings can be left in place for seven days to reduce the potential for infection, although advice from the appropriate surgical team, and/or tissue viability or medical teams, should be followed alongside manufacturers' recommendations.

Wounds caused by congenital conditions

These wounds are more likely to require special care and attention. This category includes epidermolysis bullosa (EB), a group of skin conditions where the common factor is a tendency for the skin to blister or shear away in response to minimal friction or trauma (*Chapter 10*). These mechano-bullous disorders vary in course and severity from minor disability to death in early infancy. The prevalence of severe forms of EB in the UK is approximately 1:175000 live births, and these infants require specialised handling techniques to avoid epidermal stripping as a result of friction and shearing forces (www.debra.org.uk).

The wounds should be dressed with appropriate non-adherent material, but care must be taken because many dressings described by the manufacturer as being 'non-adherent' behave differently on those affected by EB.

Products that bond to the skin, such as adhesive dressings or tapes, must be avoided and cardiac and oxygen saturation monitors fixed in place with a non-adherent dressing to prevent skin injury. In particular, soft silicone dressings can be useful as a tape for patients with EB. However, if bonding does occur, the adhesive can be dissolved using a greasy emollient white soft paraffin (WSP) and liquid paraffin (LP) 50:50 mixture, applied liberally over the dressing/tape and worked underneath, to allow the dressing/tape to be removed without damaging the skin.

Humidity and heat can increase the rate of blistering in those with EB, and blisters must be lanced or aspirated using a hypodermic needle. It is also recommended that clothing is turned inside out to avoid seams rubbing on the skin; alternatively, flat-seamed garments can be used.

Affected infants should be nursed in a cot rather than an incubator, unless medically indicated for reasons such as prematurity. Friction and adherence of nappies can cause excoriation in those with EB, but this can be avoided by cleaning the skin with WSP/LP 50:50 and lining the nappy with soft material; the easiest being a commercial nappy liner that overlaps the edges of the nappy. Peri-umbilical trauma to the skin can occur from a cord clamp in babies with EB. To avoid this, the clamp should be removed and replaced with a ligature.

Excoriation

Excoriation in the nappy area is generally caused by prolonged contact with urine-soaked material, which can be exacerbated by frequent diarrhoea, or fungal colonisation by the resident gut flora *Candida albicans* (Boiko, 2000). If colonisation by *Candida albicans* is suspected, a skin swab should be taken and anti-fungal therapy given while waiting for swab results. Topical and enteral nystatin therapy should be prescribed and continued until there are two clear swabs. If the initial swab is negative, therapy can be discontinued immediately.

Nappies should be changed frequently (every 4–6 hours), and the skin gently cleansed with warm water only. Wipes are not necessary, as they expose the pre-term infant to unnecessary chemicals, but may be used in an older infant. Alkaline soaps, or perfumed baby bath products, should be avoided for the first few weeks of a pre-term infant's life, because the skin's protective acid mantle will not yet be developed, making it vulnerable to pH alteration by these products and leaving it more prone to bacterial colonisation. The products also contain dyes and perfumes that may irritate the skin (NANN, 1997).

A layer of hydrocolloid or zinc paste, or nappy cream will serve as an effective barrier to protect the injured skin (British National Formulary [BNF], 2003). Skin barrier films can also be used but care must be taken regarding the potential for absorption of the product in newly-born premature babies. If the baby's condition is very unstable, handling should be reduced to a minimum and all care given at one time, depending on the policy of the paediatric or neonatal unit.

The causes of wound pain

It has been argued that practitioners should follow the rule that what is painful to an adult, is painful to an infant, unless proven otherwise (Anand, 2001; Saniski, 2005). The causes of wound pain in adults and, therefore, also in children, have been described by the World Union of Wound Healing Societies (WUWHS) in a consensus document (WUWHS, 2004) as being multilayered, including background, incident, procedural and operative pain, with these all being affected by psychosocial and environmental factors (*Table 11.1*). Background pain is the pain felt at rest, and is associated with the nature or cause of the wound, or unrelated medical condition. For a child, this may include issues such as dermatological conditions, wound maceration or infection. Incident pain can occur during activities such as mobilising that may cause dressing slippage. This may be particularly significant in pre-school children and infants who are continuously moving, making dressing slippage more likely. Procedural pain results from procedures such as dressing removal and application and wound cleansing. Operative pain is associated with interventions normally carried out by a specialist clinician and requires local or general anaesthetic, such as surgery or wound debridement. Post-operative pain can also be significant, particularly for an anxious child. In fact, there are many psychosocial and environmental factors that cause increased pain in children, such as fear, education, culture, past experiences, the setting, and the noise level.

Table 11.1: The causes of wound pain	
Background causes	Aetiology/nature of the wound, eg. ischaemia, burn, infection, abrasions, donor sites
Incident causes	Friction, dressing slippage, exposure of the wound to the air
Procedural causes	Dressing or tape removal, wound cleansing, dressing application, suture removal
Operative causes	Debridement
Psychological factors	Anxiety, fear, age, past experiences
Environmental factors	Noise level, distractions, comfort, timing of procedure

(Anand, 2001; WUWHS, 2004)

Assessment of pain

Pain assessment should include the assessment of the cause and severity of the pain. Visual analogue scales that use sad and happy faces have been recommended for the assessment of the severity of pain in children over five years, and numerical scales for children over the age of ten who know their numbers (Royal College of Nursing [RCN], 2002). However, for younger children, or those that have communication difficulties, different scales need to be used that consider behavioural or physiological changes (_Table 11.2_), and there are a number of scales cited in the literature (Anand, 2001; Committee on Fetus and Newborn/ Canadian Paediatric Society, 2000; RCN, 2002). The practitioner must ensure that whichever scale or tool they are using, it has been validated for use within the age group of the child, and that it is not used in isolation but that the views of the parents, the clinical condition, and context of the child are also considered (RCN, 2002).

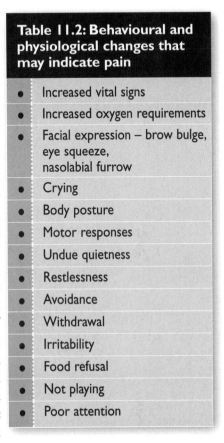

Table 11.2: Behavioural and physiological changes that may indicate pain
• Increased vital signs
• Increased oxygen requirements
• Facial expression – brow bulge, eye squeeze, nasolabial furrow
• Crying
• Body posture
• Motor responses
• Undue quietness
• Restlessness
• Avoidance
• Withdrawal
• Irritability
• Food refusal
• Not playing
• Poor attention

Anand, 2002; RCN, 2002

Pain assessment should be ongoing, not just prior to dressing changes. This will allow the practitioner to evaluate the care being provided, and detect any changes in the child's wound (Anand, 2001; Cooper _et al_, 2004).

There are a number of methods and factors that help reduce pain in paediatric wound care. These cover:

* pharmacological methods
* environmental issues
* communication with parents

- dressing procedures
- emotional/psychological factors.

Pharmacological methods

There are a variety of systemic and local analgesics that can be administered to children, and practitioners should take advice from their local pain control policies for guidance. Those commonly cited in the international literature include local anaesthetics such as EMLA (lignocaine and prilocaine hydrochloride in an emulsion base), or lignocaine and systemic analgesics, such as sucrose, paracetamol, fentanyl, opioids and non-steroidal anti-inflammatory drugs (NSAIDs) (de Lima *et al*, 1996; Committee on Fetus and Newborn/Canadian Paediatric Society, 2000; Anand, 2001; Zempsky *et al*, 2004; Saniski, 2005).

Practitioners should administer these drugs according to the results of the pain assessment. For instance, if a child is suffering from background pain, then systemic analgesics should be administered on a regular basis. If a child suffers from procedural or operative pain, then a bolus of systemic analgesic and/or local anaesthetic should be administer prior to, during, and after the procedure if necessary.

Environmental issues

Practitioner should provide non-stressful environments for dressing procedures (WUWHS, 2004). This includes preparing the room, staff, child, parents, and equipment (Committee on Fetus and Newborn/ Canadian Paediatric Society, 2000). The room should be warm and quiet; music can be played and, if practical, the light levels lowered (Saniski, 2005). No equipment should be placed on top of the incubator, even when space is limited, because of noise transmission (American Academy of Pediatrics, 1997). Non-nutritive sucking or the use of pacifiers, along with sucrose, can also be useful during a procedure (Committee on Fetus and Newborn/Canadian Paediatric Society, 2000).

Communication with parents

Parents may feel guilty or anxious that their baby has been born prematurely, or that their child might be in pain. They may need reassurance that the appropriate treatment is being carried out. It is important to identify their level of understanding and how much they want to know about their child's wound. If they wish and if it is clinically appropriate, parents should be encouraged to be involved in their infant's care. However, parents should be made aware of the procedure and their responsibilities beforehand, so that they are not surprised or shocked and inadvertently increase an infant's stress levels (Barker *et al*, 2004).

Dressing procedures

Many of the painful stimuli in wound care are caused by the dressing procedure itself, and practitioners should be aware of these painful triggers and avoid them if possible (WUWHS, 2004). Ideally, two people should assist during a dressing change, so that one is available to contain and comfort the baby, while the other changes the dressing. Dressing changes should be kept to a minimum, and tapes or dressings only removed when necessary. The dressing should be prepared before approaching or uncovering the baby, to minimise the length of time that the wound is exposed, and the baby is undressed or uncovered (Barker *et al*, 2004). This is for thermoregulatory and infection control reasons and to minimise stress.

Warm fluids should be used to wash the wound as cold fluids will reduce the temperature of the wound bed and, as a result, polymorphic and macrophagic activity will cease until the temperature increases again. Irrigation with cold fluids can also cause pain. Practitioners should avoid touching wounds unnecessarily because this can also cause pain and trauma (Cooper *et al*, 2004). To prevent cross-contamination, nursing staff should conform to the principles of aseptic technique during all dressing procedures (Darmstadt and Dinulos, 2000).

Emotional/psychological factors

The psychological factors that contribute to the child's pain, listed in *Table 11.2*, must also be addressed if they are to be managed holistically. The management of these psychological factors will depend on the age of the child.

The issues discussed above should be addressed to ensure that the environment is conducive to minimising stress. It is important for children to have a parent or family member present during the dressing procedure, so that the child has a familiar person with them (Zempsky *et al*, 2004). The parent and the child will also need reassuring to reduce their anxiety and encourage their trust and co-operation. When managing chronic wounds, it is appropriate for the parent to be taught how to apply the dressing themselves to encourage independence.

The practitioner should be taught how to reduce a child's stress by talking openly and honestly, and using language that they understand, such as 'poorly finger' (Committee on Fetus and Newborn/Canadian Paediatric Society, 2000). The amount of information that is given should be tailored to the needs and age of the child. Detailed descriptions and lengthy explanations can increase anxiety in an over-anxious child; the practitioner should assess each child individually. Reward stickers are a useful means of gaining co-operation in a primary school-aged child (Barker *et al*, 2004).

Distraction and comforting techniques should be employed, such as allowing the child to play with the dressings; applying the dressings to dolls or teddies; encouraging the child to play, read, or sing during the procedure; or using music or bubbles (Zempsky *et al*, 2004). Younger children should be swaddled or cuddled during the dressing change, and clustering care for children that are requiring a number of different interventions is useful when followed by a period of rest (Saniski, 2005).

Practitioners should negotiate with older children to come to an agreement on the plan of care, including the amount of patient involvement in the procedure, time-out breaks, and analgesia regimes (Barker *et al*, 2004).

The choice of dressing

Ideally, any wound dressing used on a paediatric patient should be able to protect the wound while being atraumatic, ie. prevent trauma and pain to the wound or surrounding skin on removal. Painful stimuli can be avoided by choosing dressings that are easy to apply, do not need to be changed too frequently, and promote wound healing (WUWHS, 2004). Where appropriate, the dressing should be cut to the correct size of the wound to prevent it coming into contact with the surrounding skin. However, in a humidified environment, there may be problems with dressings staying in place.

Non-interactive dressing products, such as soft silicone wound contact layers or hydrocolloids, hydrogels, foams and semi-permeable films, are routinely used (Darmstadt and Dinulos, 2000). If adhesive dressings, such as films or hydrocolloids, are used, these should be left in place for extended periods of time because their adhesive nature will reduce over time. Dressings that create a moist wound-healing environment encourage autolytic debridement (Miller, 2000). If surgical debridement is required, an appropriately qualified person must perform it in a controlled environment. There is limited research-based evidence to guide the selection of the most suitable products. It is important to liaise with the tissue viability team, refer to local wound management guidelines, and to contact other neonatal units to ascertain their practices.

Documentation

It is important that all wound care objectives, wound assessments and management plans are documented. A documented wound assessment should include details of (Bale and Morison, 1998):

- the type of wound
- the position of the wound
- wound dimensions (length, width and depth)
- the nature of the wound bed
- the condition of surrounding skin

- exudate level
- colour and consistency
- presence of odour and infection
- level of pain.

Conclusion

Skin and wound complications are a source of morbidity and unnecessary suffering in neonates and older paediatrics, and the appropriate prevention and management of pain should be central to the care of this vulnerable population. All healthcare practitioners have an ethical and professional obligation to ensure that paediatric pain is minimised. The prevention and management of pain and trauma associated with wound care should involve both an ongoing and comprehensive assessment of the risk factors associated with trauma and pain, and the causes of pain, including physical, psychological and environmental factors. This assessment should be followed by the implementation of a multi-faceted approach to pain management that includes environmental, pharmacological and psychological strategies, the aim being to preserve skin integrity, where possible, and to minimise trauma and pain during wound care procedures.

This chapter has been adapted from, and reproduced by kind permission of, Wounds UK 2(1): 33–41, written on behalf of The Neonatal Advisory Group: Elaine Bethell, Clinical Nurse Specialist Tissue Viability, City Hospital, Birmingham; Fiona Burton, Nurse Consultant Tissue Viability, University Hospitals Coventry and Warwickshire (UHCW) NHS Trust; Jacqueline Denyer, Clinical Nurse Specialist Epidermolysis Bullosa, Great Ormond Street Hospital for Children, London; Sandra Edwards, Neonatal Surgical Support Sister, Princess Anne Hospital, Southampton; Dr Helen Goodyear, Consultant Paediatrician, Heartlands Hospital, Birmingham; Valerie Irving, Neonatal Unit Manager, Liverpool Women's Hospital; Sooi Litchfield, Advanced Neonatal Nurse Practitioner, Neonatal Unit, University Hospitals Coventry and Warwickshire NHS Trust; Mark O'Brien, Clinical Nurse Specialist Tissue Viability, Great Ormond Street Hospital for Children, London; Fiona Smith, Royal College of Nursing, Adviser in Children's and Young People's Nursing; Debbie Tompkins, Advanced Neonatal Nurse Practitioner, City Hospital, Birmingham; Trudie Young, Lecturer in Tissue Viability, School of Nursing, University of Wales Bangor.

References

American Academy of Pediatrics (1997) Noise: A hazard for the fetus and newborn. *Pediatrics* **100**(4): 724–7

American Academy of Pediatrics/Canadian Paediatric Society (2000) Prevention and management of pain and stress in the neonate. *Pediatrics* **105**: 454–61

Anand KJ (1998) Clinical importance of pain and stress in preterm newborn neonates. *Biol Neonate* **73**(1): 1–9

Anand KJ (2001) International Evidence-Based Group for Neonatal Pain Consensus statement for the prevention and management of pain in the newborn. *Arch Pediatr Adolesc Med* **155**(2): 173–80

Association of Women's Health, Obstetric and Neonatal Nurses (2001) *Evidence-based clinical practice guideline. Neonatal Skin care.* AWHONN. Available online at: www.awhonn.org

Bale S, Morison M (1997) Patient assessment. In: Morison M, Moffatt C, Bridel-Nixon J, Bale S, eds. *Nursing Management of Chronic Wounds.* Mosby, London, Chap 4: 69–86

Barker A, Burton F, Bryan J *et al* (2004) Issues in Paediatric Wound Care, Minimising Trauma and Pain. Tendra Academy, Mölnlycke Health Care

Blatz S, Paes B (1990) Intravenous infusion by superficial vein in the neonate. *J Intravenous Nurs* **13**(2): 122–8

Boiko S (2000) Making rash decisions in the diaper area. *Pediatr Ann* **29**(1): 50–6

Bravery K (1999) Paediatric intravenous therapy in practice. In: Doughtery L, Lamb J, eds. *Intravenous Therapy in Nursing Practice.* Churchill Livingstone, London: 401–45

British National Formulary (2003) *British National Formulary.* Royal Pharmaceutical Society of Great Britain, London

Committee on Fetus and Newborn/Canadian Paediatric Society (2000) Prevention and management of pain and stress in the neonate. *Pediatrics* **105**: 454–61

Cooper P, Russell F, Stringfellow S (2004) *Best Practice Statement Minimising Trauma and Pain in Wound Management.* Issue 1. Tendra Academy, Mölnlycke Health Care. Available online at: www.wounds-uk.com

Darmstadt GL, Dinulos JG (2000) Neonatal skin care. *Pediatr Dermatol* **47**(4): 757–81

de Lima J, Lloyd-Tomas AR, Howard RF, Sumner E (1996) Infant and neonatal pain: anaesthetists' perceptions and prescribing patterns. *Br Med J* **313**: 787

Evans NJ, Rutter N (1986) Development of the epidermis in the newborn. *Biol Neonate* 49(2): 74–80

Glynn G (2004) A low technology type of device for nasal CPAP. *J Neonatal Nurs* 10(4): 108–10

Gunderson L, Kenner C (1995) *Care of the 24–25-week gestational age infant: a small baby protocol.* 2nd edn. NICU Ink, Petaluma (CA)

Hardman MJ, Moore L, Ferguson MWJ, Byrne C (1999) Barrier formation in the human fetus is patterned. *J Invest Dermatol* 113: 1106–14

Harpin V, Rutter N (1982) Percutaneous alcohol absorption and skin necrosis in a preterm infant. *Arch Dis Childhood* 57: 477–9

Hecker J (1993) Survival of neonatal intravenous infusion sites. *Int J Pharmacy Practice* 2: 82–5

Hecker J, Duffy B, Fong T, Wyer M (1991) Failure of intravenous infusions in neonates. *J Paediatr Child Health* 27: 175–9

Independent Advisory Group report (2005) Issues in Neonatal Wound Care – Minimising Trauma and Pain. Tendra Academy, Mölnlycke Health Care. Available online at: www.tendra.com

Irving V (2001a) Caring for and protecting the skin of pre-term neonates. *J Wound Care* 10(7): 253–6

Irving V (2001b) Reducing the risk of epidermal stripping in the neonatal population: an evaluation of an alcohol-free barrier film. *J Neonatal Nurs* 7(1): 5–8

Johnston CC, Stevens BJ, Franck LS, Jack A, Stremler R, Platt R (1999) Factors explaining lack of response to heel stick in preterm newborns. *J Obstet Gynecol Neonatal Nurs* 28(6): 587–94

Linder N, Davidovitch N, Reichman B *et al* (1997) Topical iodine-containing antiseptics and subclinical hypothyroidism in preterm infants. *J Pediatr* 131(3): 434–9

Lund C (1999) Prevention and management of infant skin breakdown. *Nurs Clin N Am* 34(4): 907–20

Malloy-McDonald M (1995) Skin care for high risk neonates. *J Wound Ostomy Continence Nurs* 22(4): 177–82

McManus Kuller J (2001) Skin breakdown: risk factors, prevention and treatment. *Newborn Infant Nurs Rev* 1(1): 35–42

McManus Kuller J, Lund C, Nonato LB (2002) Neonatal integumentary system. In: *Pediatrics Clinical Education Series*. Ross Products Division, Abbot Laboratories Inc

Merskey H, Bogduk N, eds (1994) *Classification of Chronic Pain.* 2nd edn. IASP Task Force on Taxonomy, IASP Press, Seattle:209–14. Available online at: www.iasp-pain.org

Miller M (2000) Moist wound healing. In: *Essential Wound Healing*, Part 1. EMAP Healthcare, London

National Association for Neonatal Nurses (1997) *Neonatal Skin Care: guidelines for practice*. NANN, California. Available online at: www. nann.org

Porter FL, Grunau RE, Anand KJ (1999) Long-term effects of pain in infants. *J Develop Behav Pediatr* **20**: 253–61

Royal College of Nursing (2002) *Clinical Practice Guidelines: The Recognition and Assessment of Acute Pain in Children. Technical Report.* RCN, London

Rutter N (1996) The immature skin. *Eur J Pediatr* **155**(suppl 2): S18–S20

Rutter N (2000) Clinical consequences of an immature barrier. *Semin Neonatol* **5**(4): 281–7

Saniski D (2005) *Neonatal pain relief protocols in their infancy*. Available online at: www.nurseweek.com, 14 February 2005

Watkins A, Keogh E (1992) Alcohol burns in the neonate. *J Paediatr Child Health* **28**: 306–8

West D, Worbec S, Solomon L (1981) Pharmacology and toxicology of infant skin. *J Invest Dermatol* **76**: 147–50

World Union of Wound Healing Societies (2004) Principles of best practice: Minimising pain at wound dressing-related procedures. A consensus document. MEP Ltd, London

Wysocki AB (2000) Anatomy and physiology of skin and soft tissue. In: Bryant AD, ed. *Acute and Chronic Wounds: Nursing management*. 2nd edn. Mosby, St Louis

Zempsky WT, Cravero JP, Committee on Pediatric Emergency Medicine and Section on Anesthesiology and Pain Medicine (2004) Relief of pain and anxiety in pediatric patients in emergency medical systems. *Pediatrics* **114**: 1348–56

CHAPTER 12

PSYCHOLOGICAL CONSIDERATIONS IN PAEDIATRIC WOUND CARE

Kristina Soon

There have been a number of developments over the last few decades in paediatric disease management that have contributed to the role of psychology becoming more prominent in this field. Firstly, scientific research has now created a body of evidence that demonstrates a clear link between physical and psychological well-being, so that psychological intervention is becoming a common component in the care of physical problems. This has happened in the context of a general move towards multidisciplinary care and a focus on holistic constructs, such as quality of life, as being ideal measures of health outcome, rather than purely medical measures. Secondly, as medical technology has improved, more people are surviving serious illness and injury, and a larger proportion of our community now live with the challenges and constraints associated with illness. Thirdly, important documents, such as The Bristol Royal Infirmary Inquiry (2001) and the National Service Frameworks (NSFs) for Children, Young People and Maternity Services (Department of Health [DoH], 2004) have highlighted the importance of patient-focused, developmentally appropriate care, in particular, services that are engineered not just to address the physical needs, but also the mental health and emotional needs of children and their families.

This chapter summarises some of the relevant literature relating to the link between psychological and physiological function, in the case of wound care in children. In the first section, the evidence for the contribution of psychological function to wound healing is described. In the second, the way in which illness can, in turn, contribute to psychological function is discussed. The final section introduces some simple ideas, which can be incorporated into paediatric wound care, that help to address some of the issues raised in the first two sections. This chapter is not intended to be an exhaustive catalogue of the different ways in which psychological and physiological factors interact in the context of paediatric wound care, but rather to describe some key areas where evidence has already been collected, and where minor changes in your work with the patient may be able to affect significant change.

How psychology can influence physiology

Baum and Posluszny (1999) described some different pathways along which psychological factors can affect physical health. One pathway is via direct biological changes that occur as part of an emotional reaction or behaviour pattern. For example, there are many studies that show that emotion-based stress responses can increase blood pressure, heart rate, and sympathetic arousal that can result in heart disease, hypertension or cardiac events. Another pathway along which psychology affects disease is through behaviours that occur in relation to the illness, such as adherence to treatment regimes and behaviours that impair healing.

A few of the pathways linking psychological function to physiological changes that are relevant to wound healing are described below. These pathways are:

- the effect of psychological factors on physiological systems
- adherence to treatment
- scratching.

The effect of psychological factors on physiological systems

There are a number of routes that have been identified as being important to the mind-body link, particularly between psychological arousal, the central nervous system, and the endocrine and immune systems. For example, stress has been shown to increase levels of certain neurotransmitters and hormones. Research has identified receptors for hormones and neurotransmitters on immunological cells, such as lymphocytes. Furthermore, there is evidence of direct nervous system influence on the immune system, such as the autonomic innervation of the thymus gland, which produces T-cells. The hypothalamus is a key structure involved with base emotional responses, such as fear, which has been shown to be strongly linked with the immune function (Siegel and Grahame-Pole, 1995). These functions have been implicated in the aetiology and progression of viral infections, wound healing, cancer and human immunodeficiency virus (HIV). Blalock (1984) has shown that immune cells, in turn, communicate with every other system in the body. Through this link, it is possible to envisage a total integration of mind and body that results in healing, or a failure to heal. A meta-analytic study of the literature regarding the link between psychological stress and immunity in humans, concluded that there was compelling evidence for a reliable association between a wide range of stressors and, at least, transient reductions in functional immune measures, such as numbers and percentages of lymphocytes, immunoglobulin levels and antibody titers to herpes viruses (Herbert and Cohen, 1993).

A number of studies have been conducted on the effect of psychological factors on wound healing, or physiological functions linked to wound healing. Broadbent *et al* (2003) found that psychological stress impaired the inflammatory response and matrix degradation processes in the wound immediately following surgery. This finding applied previous laboratory research to surgical patients and expanded the known influence of stress to connective tissue matrix remodelling processes. The authors suggested that in clinical practice, interventions to reduce the patient's psychological stress level may improve wound repair and recovery following surgery. Hashiro and Okumura (1998) investigated the relationship between psychological and immunological states of patients with atopic dermatitis. The authors concluded that high state and trait anxiety were linked to depressed immune function in their participants.

Two studies have examined the effect of psychological factors on the healing of punch biopsy wounds in healthy adults. Both found that slower healing was associated with elevated levels of stress, and lower trait optimism. None of the other health-related behaviours measured, such as alcohol intake, exercise, healthy eating and sleep predicted speed of healing as well as psychological stress (Marucha *et al*, 1998; Ebrecht *et al*, 2004).

Most of the studies in this field of research focus on adults. There are few studies, to date, investigating specific links between psychological and physiological factors in children. Boyce *et al* (1996), who focused on childhood respiratory illness, demonstrated the relationship between psychological stress and immune reactivity. In a study of children with leukaemia, Siegel and Grahame-Pole (1991) found that measures of 'daily hassles' and hopelessness were consistently predictive of disease outcome. In particular, relapse was associated with anxiety, hopelessness and daily hassles. Infection, on the other hand, was linked with depressive symptoms, hopelessness and daily hassles.

Treatment adherence

Adherence to treatment regimes for children is a major health concern. Estimates suggest that overall adherence in paediatric populations is about 50%, although this tends to worsen over time in both acute and chronic illnesses (Rapoff, 1999), and in conditions requiring complex management (Johnson, 1994). Wounds, and other dermatological conditions, are particularly challenging in that their treatments are often complex and time-consuming, requiring a great deal of skill, organisation and self-discipline. Also, treatments are often associated with physical discomfort, pain, or the unpleasant greasiness and odour of many topical treatments.

Treatment adherence has been widely researched, as it plays a key role in recovery from illness, and is a subject of concern for healthcare professionals. A number of key factors should be considered when trying to maximise adherence and, hence, recovery.

A schedule of reward and punishment related to the treatment process has been found to be important. Treatments with the poorest adherence were those where improvements were not clearly observable and, therefore, provided little reward for the behaviour of applying the treatment. Similarly, treatments that did not provide immediate positive consequences, or had variable efficacy, were adhered to poorly. Treatments that were associated with aversive side-effects, such as pain or disfigurement, were also more problematic (Litt and Cuskey, 1980). The same study also found that treatments that had long-term, rather than immediate effects, were not sufficiently motivating to improve daily behaviour. Treatments that were considered to be punishing, in that they interfered with the child's normal development or daily activities, were found to cause adherence problems (Matsui, 2000). Likewise, treatments that required significant lifestyle adjustments, altered the patient's appearance, or impaired their social interactions in some way were also linked to poorer adherence (La Greca, 1990).

A number of studies have tried to identify factors within the child patient that might contribute to poor treatment adherence. For example, Lemanek (1990) has found consistently that demographic variables, such as race, gender, religion and educational level, are not good predictors of adherence in paediatric populations.

Children described as psychologically well-adjusted were found to be better at adhering to treatment (La Greca and Bearman, 2003), and adolescent patients were found to have greater difficulties with adherence than younger children (Brownbridge and Fielding, 1994). However, adolescents were found to be better than younger children at tolerating invasive or aversive treatments (La Greca, 1990). While difficulties with treatment adherence in adolescence are often attributed to teenage 'rebelliousness', this is not borne out in the research. Instead, it is hypothesised that some of the difficulties that arise in adolescent treatment adherence are linked to factors such as reduction of parental involvement, social pressures, and increased life demands (La Greca and Bearman, 2003).

Studies have found that family factors are central in determining paediatric treatment adherence. Rapoff (1999) found that the family's adherence history was one of the most important factors to consider in disease management. Numerous studies have found an inverse relationship between family conflict and adherence in childhood illness (Hauser *et al*, 1990).

Another area that has been investigated is the relationship between patient and carers and the healthcare professionals managing the patient's care. There are a number of studies that show that clear communication between professional and patient or parents, parental satisfaction with medical care, good doctor-patient rapport, and a positive perception of the professional's supportiveness, care and empathy were all associated with improved treatment adherence (Litt and Cuskey, 1984; Ievers-Landis and Drotar, 2000). Continuity of care also saw an improvement in adherence (Litt and Cuskey, 1980).

Scratching

Scratching is a common contributor to prolonged skin healing, and most obviously occurs as an attempt to relieve an itch. However, scratching can also exacerbate the itch, leading to more scratching. Ultimately, this cycle of itching and scratching can result in significant damage to the area of skin concerned. As scratching an itch generally results in a pleasurable sensation of immediate relief, it is powerfully re-inforced. Like any behaviour that is reinforced, it becomes more frequent.

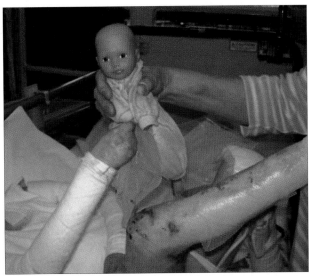

Figure 12.1: Children can be helped through painful procedures by means of distraction. This child likes her doll to help remove her dressings

Scratching can also become associated with objects, places or activities, so that these things can trigger this reaction without any purposeful intention on the part of the patient. For example, as a child relaxes in front of the television or as they listen to their teacher in class. Thus, as with many other habits, such as nail-biting, scratching can become automatic (Bridgett _et al_, 1996). Scratching can also be reinforced by the reactions of carers around the patient. For some vulnerable children, scratching becomes a powerful means of attracting the notice of their parents or carers. Although the attention they attract tends to be negative, in the form of scolding or punishment, for some children, negative attention is preferable to no attention at all.

In a small number of patients with skin complaints, wound healing may be prolonged in a purposeful way by either the patient, or a carer of the patient. It is also the case that there are some patients whose wounds are caused deliberately. This type of behaviour is now called 'fabricated and induced illness'. It is important to discriminate between patients who fall into the category of a habit-related or scratching behaviour, whose actions impede wound healing, but as an unwanted side-effect of the behaviour, to patients where the behaviours occur primarily for the purpose of worsening or creating wounds for the sake of engaging the support of professionals and others in their social network.

How physical illness can cause psychological problems

Wounds can be part of a chronic or acute condition. However, both short- and long-term illnesses, and the consequent exposure to medical procedures, have been shown to affect psychological adjustment in children. For example, up to 11% of children experience significant behaviour disturbance within two weeks of surgery (Lumley *et al*, 1993), and as many as 93% of pre-school children display increased anxiety and/or aggression after hospitalisation or minor medical procedures. Many researchers have conceptualised the experience of illness or injury in childhood as a major, stressful life event, alongside others such as family breakdown, exposure to violence, natural disasters and persistent poverty. Experience of such stressors has commonly been associated with both internalising and externalising problems such as depression, anxiety and aggression (Margolin and Gordis, 2000).

Several, large-scale studies have provided data on the effects of illness on the psychological adjustment in children. Lavigne and Faier-Routman (1992) conducted a meta-analysis of over 700 studies. Their conclusion was that children with physical illnesses were approximately twice as likely to experience adjustment difficulties than their healthy peers. There was also some evidence to suggest that these children were more likely to experience internalising disorders, such as anxiety, rather than externalising disorders, such as conduct disorders, and that they were more likely to have poor self-esteem and self-concept, although these factors were linked to race, socio-economic background, ethnic background and age. Bennett (1994) conducted a meta-analysis of studies of depression among children with medical problems. He concluded that children with illnesses were at an increased risk of developing clinical depression, as well as sub-clinical depressive symptomatology.

There are a number of ways in which physical illness can lead to psychological difficulties. A few of these pathways are described below. These are:

- pain and distress related to medical procedures
- difficulties with peer relationship
- disfigurement
- changes in family dynamics.

Pain and distress related to medical procedures

Many studies show that the pain and emotional distress that occur in relation to medical procedures, major and minor, can have both short- and long-term consequences on child patients. Not only can the child become emotionally stressed, but he/she can also become reluctant to engage in later medical procedures, which can have major consequences on their carers and on their own psychological and physical health in the long term. Management of skin conditions is typically characterised by regular treatments, which can become the source of ongoing and escalating distress for the child and their family.

A number of different causes of emotional distress in children have been hypothesised, such as: actual pain; anticipation of pain; fear of embarrassment through screaming or crying; fear of being physically restrained; fear of failing to tolerate the procedure; fear of disappointing parents or professionals; fear of being punished for failing; and fear of feeling fearful. Thus, the distress may not be related directly to the procedure, but to factors that have become related to it. The pain and distress associated with a specific medical procedure can then be generalised to other benign things which the child associates with the procedure, such as the professional administering the treatment, the setting, or the equipment used. These 'paired associations' can cause significant obstructions to later procedures.

Some studies have attempted to identify factors that might contribute to the experience of high levels of distress in response to medical procedures. Lee and White-Traut (1996) found temperament to be predictive of distress. Children who were highly emotional, or not as adaptable as their peers, tended to experience more distress. A number of studies, such as Rudolph *et al* (1995), have also reported that distress in previous procedures, predicted distress in future procedures, contradicting the commonly held belief that children will spontaneously tolerate procedures better over time, or that children who have had many procedures before will cope better. The same study found that it was not clear if there was a difference between boys and girls in the amount of distress experienced. However, younger children tended to give higher pain intensity ratings than older children, and to exhibit more overt distress. Researchers have also shown that parent behaviour in the treatment room can account for up to 53% of the variance in child distress behaviour (Frank *et al*, 1995), highlighting the importance of preparing the parents as much as the child.

While the immediate pain and distress related to a medical procedure is normally observable, there can also be long-term physiological and psychological consequences that are less noticeable to the professionals involved in the child's care. Ruda *et al* (2000) suggested that early pain experiences can permanently alter neuronal connections that process pain in the spinal cord. For example, babies circumcised without anaesthesia, compared to uncircumcised babies and babies circumcised with anaesthesia, showed accentuated behavioural responses to immunisations at 4–6 months of age (Taddio *et al*, 1997). Reports of pain and fear from medical procedures in childhood is also highly predictive of pain and fear of medical procedures, and avoidance of medical care in young adulthood (Pate *et al*, 1996).

There is also evidence to show that emotional distress, such as elevated anxiety, general upset, anger and low mood can increase a person's pain perception (McGrath, 1994), rendering each subsequent procedure more painful and fear-provoking. Without adequate pain management and emotional containment early in the medical experience, aversive medical procedures are likely to result in a cycle of pain, distress, conditioned anticipatory anxiety, and more pain (Choiniere, 2001).

Difficulties with peer relationships

A substantial amount of research has investigated the role of peer relationships in the social and emotional development of children. These studies consistently find that positive peer relationships in childhood lead to positive psychological and social outcomes in later life (Reiter-Pertill and Noll, 2003). Children with good friendship links generally feel better about themselves and perform better academically, while those with poor peer relationships not only perform less well at school, but also tend to have more behavioural difficulties. Good peer relationships are a strong predictor of positive adaptation to secondary school in children with chronic illness. Similarly, socially isolated behaviour is a risk factor predictive of future problems with social acceptance by peers, negative self-perceptions, anxiety and depression (Hymel *et al*, 1990).

La Greca (1990) has suggested several characteristics of diseases and/or treatments that might affect a child's peer relationships. Firstly, there is the restriction in physical activities or interference with daily activities, including school attendance, that may result in a child being less able or less available to participate in peer-oriented activities. Secondly, changes in physical appearance lead to negative self-perception or negative reactions from peers. Finally, cognitive impairment, resulting from illness or treatment, is likely to lead to difficulties in peer relationships.

There are certainly a number of studies that suggest that children with illness are more likely to be rated as socially withdrawn, lonely, shy, having poorer social skills, and more school absences. For example, in a study of children with neurofibromatosis, parents and teachers rated these children as having more social problems, being more withdrawn with less social competence than their healthy peers (Johnson *et al*, 1999).

Disfigurement

As with other aspects of psychological adjustment to medical problems, having a disfiguring condition or wound does not necessarily cause the affected person to have psychological difficulties. However, the research is clear that children who look different are at greater risk of suffering from psychological and social difficulties (Walters, 1997). Interestingly, some obvious features of disfigurement that might appear to influence psychological adjustment, such as the severity and visibility of the disfigurement, are not strong predictors of psychological outcome (Knudson-Cooper, 1981).

Psychological difficulties can occur for a number of different reasons. In the case of children who look different from birth, Langlois and Sawin (1981) found that such babies were held less closely by their parents, and given less ventral contact than babies with normal appearance. This could affect the early interaction and relationship between parent and child, at a crucial time when the baby is learning the fundamental rules of interpersonal relationships.

Pertschuk and Whitaker (1987 in Landsdowne) reported that children who look different are more likely to experience clinically significant levels of anxiety. They are also more likely to withdraw socially and avoid situations where they might meet new people, which can prevent these children from developing their social skills and confidence (Walters, 1997). There is some evidence that children who look different are more likely to exhibit behavioural problems.

Older children, in particular, are more likely than their healthy peers to exhibit disruptive and uncooperative behaviour. One hypothesis is that eliciting negative responses from people around them for bad behaviour is a means of avoiding or pre-empting negative responses about their appearance (Walters, 1997).

Changes in family dynamics

One of the key factors that differentiates paediatric working to adult care is that the child patient is always embedded within a family system, whether it be their biological, nuclear family, or another arrangement of carers. This can be an advantage in that there are a number of people who can assist in managing the medical condition. However, these extra people must also be considered in terms of how they are coping with the medical condition and treatment demands, and the way in which they affect disease management and the well-being of the child.

Wood (1994) concluded that the family was probably the single most influential factor in the lives of children with illness and, as such, it is important to consider family interactions as psychophysiological mediators of stress.

There have been a number of studies that have identified common stresses in the life of a family with a sick member. These include strained family relationships, limitations on family activities and goals, increased tasks and time commitments, financial burdens, housing adaptation, social isolation, concerns about medical care, ie. competence, altered educational experience and grief (Altschuler, 1997). Prolonged responsibility for disease management can also regulate and restrict relationships between family members. The restrictions that parents must enforce as part of a treatment regime can alter relationships, from having to impose strict routines to crossing physical boundaries, such as having to see an older child naked in order to complete skin care regimes. Faced with an illness, the family has to adapt to considerable change in roles, structure, and patterns of relating. How these changes are integrated is determined by both the beliefs of the family and its organisation. A family's responses are also affected by personal resources, physical and emotional energy, intellect, confidence, threshold for stress and coping styles.

Of course, families are not just affected by illness within their midst, but can influence the progress of the illness in return. Wood

(1994) described three key potential inter-relational difficulties within families with a sick child, namely:

* A close family with particularly strong or weak generational boundaries was linked with high emotionality in relation to medical challenges.
* A situation of triangulation, where a parent teams up with a child against the other parent, or parents express their own conflict through the child, has been associated with greater disease activity (Woods *et al*, 1989), and with stress-related physiological arousal in the child (Gottman and Fainsilber Katz, 1989).
* A family that is emotionally distant, where parents do not take appropriate and helpful control and responsibility is likely to leave a sick child vulnerable. This type of family structure may undermine medical compliance and fail to protect a child from stresses.

Conclusion

Without doubt, research that describes and demonstrates the link between physiological and psychological function is becoming quite substantial. There is good evidence to suggest that, in the field of paediatric wound care, psychological factors can be the cause of complications in the healing process and that they can be caused by the consequences of having a wound and its related medical treatments. On the basis of the research evidence, the final section of this chapter outlines some simple ideas to incorporate into your daily practice that can help to minimise the effects of the psychology-physiology links described above. However, significant and unremitting concerns about psychological well-being should always be referred on to appropriately qualified mental health professionals.

Things to do in day-to-day practice...

While research is still in its early stages, the most promising developments in helping children to tolerate medical experiences are, fortunately, linked to factors referred to as proximal variables. These include the behaviour of the adults, children's knowledge, thoughts, memories and coping behaviours, and decreasing pain and the nature of the procedure itself (Blount *et al*, 2003). Distal variables, such as personality, age, temperament and other trait-like variables, do not appear to be useful *foci* when helping children to tolerate distressing procedures better.

Reducing psychological stress/adjustment

❖ Be vigilant of signs of emotional, behavioural and relational problems in the child patient and their family, as compared to their pre-morbid function, or in comparison to children of the same age and other families.

❖ Explain to parents or carers early on that psychological difficulties can occur as a result of medical problems. This can help to normalise the difficulties if they occur, and allow them to respond rapidly and constructively.

❖ Ask the patient and their family about levels and sources of daily stress, and work with them to minimise the stressors as far as possible. Encourage a sense of hope in the patient and their carers.

❖ Identify sources of social support and help the family to maximise their own coping strategies to deal with both medical and psychological difficulties.

❖ Explain the condition and treatment clearly to the child, in language appropriate to their age. Keeping the patient informed can reduce stress from uncertainty, and facilitate positive coping mechanisms.

Treatment adherence

❖ Adopt realistic expectations and accept that families must be allowed to decide how to balance healthcare needs with the need to achieve normal social and emotional function for their child.

❖ Always view the child patient and the family as active participants in the medical decision-making process, and give them as much choice and flexibility as possible.

❖ Ensure that the treatment process is engineered to disrupt the child's daily life, interests and priorities as little as possible.

❖ Where there are high levels of conflict or confusion around responsibility for care, help the family devise a collaborative approach towards treatment. This may involve, for example, helping them to write a contract or timetable clearly stating each person's duties in relation to the treatment process.

❖ Remain mindful of the reinforcement schedule relating to the treatment. Overall, it is important to try to make the experience as rewarding as possible. This might involve minimising inherently punishing aspects of treatment, such as pain, and increasing reinforcement, for example, by establishing a formal reward system, or ensuring that carers remember to be positive and praise the child's cooperation and behaviour during treatment.

❖ Maintaining a positive, communicative and supportive relationship between professional team and patient and family should be a priority.

Scratching

❖ Minimise itchiness as much as possible.

❖ Establish behavioural strategies to replace scratching with a behaviour that provides some physical relief for itching, such as by pinching or slapping the itchy area, or by applying a cold compress.

❖ In the case of automatic scratching, the patient needs to become aware of when they are scratching via a monitoring process. This should be a process that does not become punitive for the child. Once the child is more aware of when they are scratching, or the circumstances when they are at risk of scratching, alternative behaviours can be substituted.

❖ See 'Atopic Skin Disease: A manual for practitioners' by Bridgett, Noren and Staughton (1996) for more ideas for stopping scratching.

Pain and distress

* Do not assume that distress at medical procedures will decrease spontaneously over time.
* Work collaboratively with the child and family to identify specific aspects of the treatment process, or the medical condition, that cause pain and distress, and minimise them as soon as possible.
* Help the child to feel in control of medical procedures by giving them choices in how things happen.
* Try to make the experience as enjoyable as possible.
* Pain control should be considered even in minor procedures. Use of analgesia, or behavioural pain management techniques, such as distraction and relaxation, should be used in all potentially painful procedures.

Disfigurement

* Dressings can be minimised or decorated to be more acceptable to the patient and to other people who might see the dressings.
* Wounds should be made to look as unthreatening as possible so as not to upset the child or other people who might see them.
* Underlying and persistent psychological problems, such as low self-worth and social anxiety should be referred to a child mental health worker for focused intervention.

Peer relationships

* If the child is likely to come into contact with people who are not aware of their skin condition, such as at school, the child should be prepared with a few standard answers for questions about their skin, or ways of responding if they are stared at.
* The skin condition should be explained to people involved in the child's daily life, such as school teachers and the patient's friends and their parents. This can put to rest any concerns that others may have about the nature of the skin problem.
* The family should be encouraged to maintain peer-related activities and contacts.

Looking after the family

❖ The psychological well-being of the rest of the family should also be monitored. This is helpful to the family members, but also safeguards the dependent child's well-being.
❖ Families should be encouraged to ensure that routines and positive family interactions are maintained as much as possible.

References

Altschuler J (1997) *Working with Chronic Illness: A Family Approach.* Palgrave, Hampshire

Augustin M, Maier K (2003) Psychosomatic aspects of chronic wounds. *Dermatol Psychosom* 4(1): 5–13

Baum A, Posluszny D (1999) Health Psychology: Mapping biobehavioural contributions to health and illness. *Annu Rev Psychol* 50: 137–63

Bennett D (1994) Depression among children with chronic medical problems: A meta-analysis. *J Paediatr Psychol* 19: 149–69

Blalock J (1984) The immune system as a sensory organ. *J Immunol* 132: 1067–70

Blount R, Piira T, Cohen L (2003) Management of paediatric pain and distress due to medical procedures. In: Roberts M, ed. *Handbook of Paediatric Psychology.* 3rd edn. Guilford Press, New York: 216–33

Boyce W, Chesney M, Alkon A, Tschann J, Adam S, Chesterman B *et al* (1996) Psychobiological reactivity to stress and childhood respiratory illness: results of two prospective studies. *Psychosom Med* 58(4): 392–3

Bridgett C, Noren P, Staughton R (1996) *Atopic Skin Disease: A Manual for Practitioners.* Wrightson Biomedical Publishing Ltd, Petersfield

Bristol Royal Infirmary Inquiry (2001) Learning from Bristol: the Report of the Public Inquiry into Children's Heart Surgery at the Bristol Royal Infirmary 1984–1995. Cm 5207. July. Stationery Office, London. Available online at: www.bristol-inquiry.org.uk

Broadbent E, Petrie K, Alley P, Booth R (2003) Psychological stress impairs early wound repair following surgery. *Psychosom Med* 65: 865–9

Brownbridge G, Fielding D (1994). Psychosocial adjustment and adherence to dialysis treatment regimens. *Paediatr Nephrol* 8: 744–9

Choiniere M (2001) Burn pain: A unique challenge. *Pain: Clinical Updates* 7: 1–4

Ebrecht M, Hextall J, Kirtley L, Taylor A, Dyson M, Weinman J (2004) Perceived stress and cortisol levels predict speed of wound healing in healthy male adults. *Psychoneuroendocrinology* 29(6): 798–809

Frank N, Blount R, Smith A, Manimala N, Martin J (1995) Parent and staff behaviour, previous child medical experience and maternal anxiety as they relate to child procedural distress and coping. *J Paediatr Psychol* 20: 277–89

Gottman J, Fainsilber Katz L (1989) Effects of marital discord on children's peer interaction and health. *Dev Psychol* 25: 373–81

Hashiro M, Okumura M (1998) The relationship between the psychological and immunological state of patients with atopic dermatitis. *J Dermatol Sci* 16(3): 231–5

Hauser S, Jacobsen A, Lavori P, Wolfsdorf J, Herkowitz R, Milley J et al (1990) Adherence amongst children and adolescents with insulin-dependent diabetes mellitus over a four-year longitudinal follow-up: II. Immediate and long-term linkages with the family milieu. *J Paediatr Psychol* 15: 527–42

Herbert T, Cohen S (1993) Stress and immunity in humans: A meta-analytic review. *Psychosom Med* 55: 364–79

Hymel S, Rubin K, Rowden L, Lemare L (1990) Children's peer relationships: Longitudinal predictions of internalizing and externalizing problems from middle childhood. *Child Development* 61: 2004–21

Ievers-Landis C, Drotar D (2000) Parental and child knowledge of the treatment regimen for childhood chronic illnesses: Related factors and adherence to treatment. In: Drotar D, ed. *Promoting Adherence to Medical Treatment in Childhood Chronic Illness: Concepts, methods and interventions.* Erlbaum, Mahwah, NJ: 259–82

Johnson SB (1994) Health behaviour and health status: concepts, methods and applications. *J Paediatr Psychol* 19: 129–41

Johnson S, Saal H, Lovell A, Schorry E (1999) Social and emotional problems in children with neurofibromatosis type 1: Evidence and proposed interventions. *J Paediatr* 134: 767–72

Knudson-Cooper M (1981) Adjustment of visible stigma, the case of a severely burned child. *Soc Sci Med* 15: 31–44

Langlois J, Sawin D (1981) *Infant physical attractiveness as an elicitor of differential parenting behaviours.* Paper presented at The Society for Research in Child Development, Boston

La Greca A (1990) Social consequences of paediatric conditions: Fertile area for future investigation and intervention? *J Paediatr Psychol* 15: 285–308

La Greca A, Bearman M (2003) Adherence to paediatric treatment regimens. In: Roberts M, ed. *Handbook of Paediatric Psychology*. 3rd edn. Guilford Press, New York: 119–41

Lavigne J, Faier-Routman J (1992) Correlates of psychological adjustment to paediatric physical disorders: A meta-analytic review and comparison with existing models. *J Dev Behav Paediatr* 14: 117–23

Lee L, White-Traut R (1996) The role of temperament in paediatric pain response. *Compre Issues Paediatr Nurs* 19: 49–63

Lemanek K (1990) Adherence issues in the medical management of asthma. *J Paediatr Psychol* 15: 437–58

Litt L, Cuskey W (1980) Compliance with medical regimens during adolescence. *Paediatr Clin N Am* 27: 1–15

Litt L, Cuskey W (1984) Satisfaction with health care: A predictor of adolescents' appointment keeping. *J Adolesc Healthcare* 5: 196–200

Lumley M, Melamed B, Abeles L (1993) Predicting children's pre-surgical anxiety and subsequent behaviour changes. *J Paediatr Psychol* 18: 481–97

Margolin G, Gordis E (2000) The effects of family and community violence on children. *Ann Rev Psychol* 51: 445–79

Marucha P, Kiecolt-Glaser J, Favegehi M (1998) Mucosal wound healing is impaired by examination stress. *Psychosom Med* 60(3): 362–5

Matsui D (2000) Children's adherence to medication treatment. In: Drotar D, ed. *Promoting Adherence to Medical Treatment in Childhood Chronic Illness: Concepts, methods and interventions*. Mahwah, Erlbaum, NJ: 135–52

McGrath P (1994) Psychological aspects of pain perception. *Arch Oral Biol* 39: 55–62

Pate J, Blount R, Cohen L, Smith A (1996) Chilhood medical experience and temperament as predictors of adult functioning in medical situations. *Children's Health Care* 25: 281–96

Pertschuk M, Whitaker L (1987) Psychosocial considerations in craniofacial deformity. *Clin Plast Surg* 14: 163–8

Reiter-Pertill J, Noll R (2003) Peer relationships of children with chronic illness. In: Roberts M, ed. *Handbook of Paediatric Psychology*. 3rd edn. Guilford Press, New York: 176–97

Rapoff M (1999) *Adherence to Paediatric Medical Regimens*. Kluwer Academic, New York

Ruda M, Ling Q, Hohmann A, Peng Y, Tachibana T (2000) Altered nocioceptive neuronal circuits after neonatal peripheral inflammation. *Science* 289: 628–631

Rudolph K, Dennig M, Weisz J (1995) Determinants and consequences of children's coping in the medical setting: Conceptualisation, review and critique. *Psychological Bull* 118: 328–57

Siegel L, Grahame-Pole J (1995) Psychoneuroimmunology. In: Roberts M, ed. *Handbook of Paediatric Psychology*. 3rd edn. Guilford Press, New York: 759–73

Taddio A, Katz J, Ilersich A, Koren G (1997) Effect of neonatal circumcision on pain response during subsequent routine vaccination. *Lancet* **349**: 599–603

Walters E (1997) Problems faced by children and families living with visible differences. In: Landsdown R, Rumsey N, Bradbury E, Carr T, Partridge J, eds. *Visibly Different: Coping with disfigurement*. Butterworth-Heinemann, Oxford: 112–20

Wood B, Watkins J Nogueira J, Zimand E, Carroll L (1989) The 'psychosomatic family': a theoretical and empirical analysis. *Family Process* **28**: 399–417

Wood B (1994) One articulation of the structural family therapy model: a biobehavioural family model of chronic illness in children. *J Fam Therapy* **16**: 53–72

INDEX

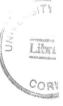